Medical Statistics at a Glance Workbook

This title is also available as an e-book.
For more details, please see
www.wiley.com/buy/9780470658482
or scan this QR code:

Companion website

Additional resources are available at:

www.medstatsaag.com

featuring:
- Excel datasets to accompany the data analysis sections
- Downloadable PDFs of two analysis templates
- Links to online further reading
- Supplementary MCQs

Medical Statistics at a Glance Workbook

Aviva Petrie

Head of Biostatistics Unit and Senior Lecturer
UCL Eastman Dental Institute
256 Grays Inn Road
London WC1X 8LD *and*
Honorary Lecturer in Medical Statistics
Medical Statistics Unit
London School of Hygiene and Tropical Medicine
Keppel Street
London WC1E 7HT

Caroline Sabin

Professor of Medical Statistics and Epidemiology
Research Department of Infection and Population Health
Division of Population Health
University College London
Royal Free Campus
Rowland Hill Street
London NW3 2PF

WILEY-BLACKWELL

A John Wiley & Sons, Ltd., Publication

This edition first published 2013 © 2013 by Aviva Petrie and Caroline Sabin

Wiley-Blackwell is an imprint of John Wiley & Sons, formed by the merger of Wiley's global Scientific, Technical and Medical business with Blackwell Publishing.

Registered office: John Wiley & Sons, Ltd, The Atrium, Southern Gate, Chichester, West Sussex, PO19 8SQ, UK

Editorial offices: 9600 Garsington Road, Oxford, OX4 2DQ, UK
The Atrium, Southern Gate, Chichester, West Sussex, PO19 8SQ, UK
111 River Street, Hoboken, NJ 07030-5774, USA

For details of our global editorial offices, for customer services and for information about how to apply for permission to reuse the copyright material in this book please see our website at www.wiley.com/wiley-blackwell.

Library of Congress Cataloging-in-Publication Data

Petrie, Aviva.
    Medical statistics at a glance workbook / Aviva Petrie, Caroline Sabin.
        p. cm.
    Includes bibliographical references and index.
    ISBN 978-0-470-65848-2 (pbk. : alk. paper)   1. Medical statistics.   I. Sabin, Caroline.
II. Title.
    R853.S7P4762 2013
    610.72'7–dc23
                                        2012025027

A catalogue record for this book is available from the British Library.

Wiley also publishes its books in a variety of electronic formats. Some content that appears in print may not be available in electronic books.

Cover design by Nathan Harris

Set in 9/11.5 pt Times by Toppan Best-set Premedia Limited

Printed and bound by CPI Group (UK) Ltd, Croydon, CR0 4YY

C9780470658482_171123

Contents

Introduction 6

Part 1: Multiple-choice questions 8
Handling data 8
Sampling and estimation 10
Study design 11
Hypothesis testing 13
Basic techniques for analysing data 13
Additional techniques 20

Part 2: Structured questions 24

Part 3: Critical appraisal 44
Randomised controlled trial: template 44
Randomised controlled trial: Paper 1 46
Observational study: template 51
Observational study: Paper 2 53

Part 4: Data analysis 61
Dataset 1 analysed by Stata v11 (StataCorp LP, Texas, USA) 61
Dataset 2 analysed using IBM SPSS Statistics v20 70

Part 5: Solutions 76
Solutions to multiple-choice questions 76
Model answers for structured questions 93
Randomised controlled trial: critical appraisal of Paper 1 109
Observational study: critical appraisal of Paper 2 113

Appendices 117
Appendix I: list of multiple-choice questions with relevant chapter numbers from *Medical Statistics at a Glance* (3rd edn) and associated topics 117
Appendix II: list of structured questions with relevant chapter numbers from *Medical Statistics at a Glance* (3rd edn) and associated topics 119
Appendix III: chapter numbers from *Medical Statistics at a Glance* (3rd edn) with relevant multiple-choice questions and structured questions 120

Companion website

Additional resources are available at:

www.medstatsaag.com

featuring:
- Excel datasets to accompany the data analysis sections
- Downloadable PDFs of two analysis templates
- Links to online further reading
- Supplementary MCQs

Introduction

This workbook is a companion volume to the third edition of *Medical Statistics at a Glance*. Although primarily directed at undergraduate medical students preparing for statistics examinations, we believe that the workbook will also be of use to others working in the biomedical disciplines who simply want to brush up on their analytical and interpretation skills (e.g. other medical researchers, postgraduates in the biomedical disciplines and pharmaceutical industry personnel). Our aim for this workbook is therefore for it to act as a revision aid, equip readers with the skills necessary to read and interpret the published literature and give them the confidence to tackle their own statistical analyses. Although designed as an accompanying text to *Medical Statistics at a Glance*, it is not indelibly linked to it and can be used as a stand-alone text or in conjunction with any reputable text on statistics.

We believe that the optimal way to learn statistics is to put the theory into practice by undertaking an analysis of a data set, but recognise that this may not always be practical. Instead, the use of carefully constructed exercises in a variety of formats can help to test and fully evaluate the reader's understanding of the material (and identify any gaps that remain). As the *At a Glance* textbook presents information in a concise manner, there is limited space in it for worked examples and no room for exercises. Our workbook amends this insufficiency by providing an extensive set of questions, as well as templates for critical appraisal and descriptions of the statistical analyses of two data sets. Where possible, we have based questions on published studies in the medical and dental fields, and references are provided so that the reader may consult the original source material if interested.

The structure of the workbook

This workbook is divided into six parts:

Part 1

This section of the workbook contains multiple-choice questions (MCQs) that are generally brief, each testing the reader's knowledge of a single theoretical concept or aspect of study interpretation. Only one of the five possible answers provided is correct: an explanation is given in Part 5 for each correct and incorrect answer. The ordering of the MCQs generally follows that of the chapters in the third edition of *Medical Statistics at a Glance*. To aid readers who may wish to focus on specific topics in the *At a Glance* textbook, we provide a list of MCQs and the related chapters in Appendix I.

Part 2

This section of the workbook contains structured questions that are longer than the MCQs and provide a more in-depth exploration of the reader's knowledge of several statistical concepts. The questions may include elements that test a reader's understanding of the theory, as well as his or her ability to interpret study findings and, in some instances, to perform basic statistical calculations. The questions are similar to those that we have set in the past for exams: detailed model answers are provided in Part 5. As the longer structured questions may relate to information contained in several diverse chapters of the textbook, these do not follow any particular order, but in Appendix II, to aid readers who may

wish to focus on specific topics in the *At a Glance* textbook, we provide a list of the structured questions and their related chapters.

Part 3

The ability to critically appraise the published literature is an essential skill that is required by anyone in the medical and dental professions (or, indeed, anyone involved in research more generally) and, consequently, is an important objective of a statistics course. Many aspects of statistics must be considered when evaluating the evidence provided in a research article, for example biases that might arise from inappropriate designs, sample size, outcome measures, the choice of statistical analysis, the presentation of the data and the conclusions drawn. Whilst *Medical Statistics at a Glance* presents a brief introduction to critical appraisal in Chapter 40 (Evidence-based medicine), Part 3 of our workbook supplements this by providing structured templates that can be used when reviewing and/or assessing the published literature. We suggest that the reader use these templates to critically appraise two published articles: a randomised controlled trial and an observational study. Our own evaluation of these articles is to be found in Part 5. Whilst we cannot hope to cover all possible topics within these two appraisals, we hope that they will at least provide a basic structure for appraisal that readers may find helpful.

Part 4

In our experience, one of the most common complaints from our students and junior research colleagues is that they just do not know where to start when analysing a substantial data set. To address this need, we have included in Part 4 a detailed description of the analyses of two data sets, the latter being available on the accompanying website (www.medstatsaag.com) as Excel files. Each analysis starts with a description of the clinical problem, and then takes the reader through the various steps that would be undertaken when performing the analysis, from the initial exploratory and descriptive analyses to the final sensitivity analyses that assess the robustness of study findings. We believe that this is an innovative approach and hope that readers will find it useful.

Part 5

This section of the workbook contains solutions to the MCQs in Part 1, model answers for the structured questions in Part 2, and our own critical appraisals of the randomised controlled trial (Paper 1) and the observational study (Paper 2) in Part 3. The pages in Part 5 are shaded so that the reader is easily able to navigate to the solutions and model answers.

Appendices

In Appendix I, we provide an ordered list of the MCQs and show which chapters they relate to, with an indication of the material included in each question. Appendix II is similar but identifies the associated chapters for the structured questions. For those readers who require exercises that relate to specific chapters of the *At a Glance* textbook, we provide a list of the chapters and indicate which multiple-choice and structured questions are relevant to them in Appendix III.

Further information

In addition to the workbook, we remind readers that the companion website to *Medical Statistics at a Glance* (www.medstatsaag.com) also contains an extensive set of interactive exercises, with references to many published papers that may be of interest.

Acknowledgements

Special thanks are due to Drs Laura Silveira-Moriyama and Angus Pringle who very kindly lent us their data sets for the analyses in Part 4 of the workbook. We are most appreciative of the extremely helpful comments and suggestions that they made during the development of the analyses, but we take full responsibility for any errors or misconceptions in the final presentations. We are also indebted to the authors and publishers of the two papers that we used for critical appraisal for allowing us to reproduce the articles, thereby providing useful exercises for our readers, and apologise if any of our criticisms cause offence. We acknowledge the generosity of the many authors and publishers who have kindly assented to our adapting or reproducing material for the multiple-choice and structured questions, and are grateful to the publishing team at Wiley-Blackwell both for suggesting that we write this workbook and for their ideas and support along its route to publication. Our acknowledgements would not be complete without thanking our students over the years from whom we have learnt the art of teaching, and Mike, Gerald, Nina, Andrew and Karen for their forbearance, encouragement and good humour during our absorption with this manuscript.

Part 1: Multiple-choice questions

Handling data

M1

To collect information on an individual's ability to function physically, investigators identified six daily tasks, each relating to a different aspect of physical functioning. For every task, respondents were asked to say whether they generally experienced 'no problems' (allocated a score of 0), 'some problems' (score of 1) or 'many problems' (score of 2) when performing the task; by summing the six individual scores, the investigators generated a total physical functioning score variable, which ranged from 0 to 12. Which one of the following statements is true?

a) The variable is best described as a continuous variable.

b) When capturing data on this score, only the final total score should be recorded on the data capture form.

c) Although this is strictly an ordinal categorical variable, for the purposes of analysis, it may be possible to treat this variable as a numerical variable.

d) The most suitable summary measure of the 'average' value for this variable would be the mode.

e) For the purposes of analysis, it would be preferable to re-categorise this final score into three categories: good functioning (scores of 0 to 4), average functioning (scores of 5 to 8) and poor functioning (scores of 9 to 12).

M2

Which one of the following statements is true?

a) A qualitative variable comprises two categories which may be ordinal or numerical.

b) An ordinal variable comprises categories which cannot be ordered.

c) The age groups 'young', 'middle aged' and 'old' relate to a nominal categorical variable.

d) Blood group is classified as a nominal categorical variable.

e) It may be difficult to distinguish a continuous numerical variable from an ordinal variable when the ordinal variable has many categories.

M3

As part of an epidemiological study investigating the association between consumption of dairy products in adolescence and the onset of cardiovascular disease later in life, study investigators plan to collect information on weekly egg consumption from a sample of children aged 14–17 years using self-administered questionnaires. Which one of the following would be the best approach for collecting this information?

a) Respondents are asked to indicate the number of eggs they consumed in the previous week and are asked to leave the entry blank if they do not know the answer.

b) Respondents are asked to tick the box that best describes the number of eggs they have consumed in the previous week: 0, 1–3, 4–7, >7 or 'unknown'.

c) Respondents are asked to indicate the number of eggs they consumed in the previous week, and to record a value of 9 if they do not know the answer.

d) Respondents are asked to tick the box that best describes the number of eggs they consumed in the previous week: 0, 1–3, 4–7 or >7; if they do not know the answer, they are asked to leave the response blank.

e) Respondents are asked to indicate the number of eggs they consumed in the previous week, and to record a value of 999 if they do not know the answer.

M4

Which one of the following statements which relate to the information provided in a questionnaire is true?

a) Having data available as an ASCII file is inflexible because many people have not heard of ASCII.

b) A multi-coded question has more than two possible responses, but the respondent can provide only one answer to it.

c) Dates must be entered into a computer spreadsheet as day/month/year.

d) Missing data for a particular respondent must always be entered on the computer spreadsheet as 9, 99 or 999.

e) It is often necessary to assign numerical codes to a categorical variable before entering the data into the computer.

M5

The number of eggs consumed by an adolescent in a week was collected from a sample of 40 adolescents aged 14–17 years with a view to estimating average weekly egg consumption in such adolescents. Information on egg consumption was missing for two adolescents; the data from the remaining 38 subjects are as follows: 0, 0, 0, 0, 0, 0, 0, 0, 0, 0, 1, 1, 1, 1, 1, 1, 1, 1, 2, 2, 2, 2, 2, 3, 3, 4, 5, 7, 7, 7, 8, 11, 14, 15, 21, 25, 27 and 71. Which one of the statements below is true?

a) The entry of 71 is an outlier but is likely to be a correct value of weekly egg consumption.

b) As it is unlikely that any individual will consume more than three eggs per day, the investigators should exclude any values greater than 21 before analysing the data.

c) As it is unlikely that any individual will consume more than three eggs per day, the investigators should replace any values >21 with the value 21 before analysing the data.

d) The authors suspect that the value of 71 is a typing error in the data set and so plan to replace this value with the value 9 before conducting any analyses.

e) The authors believe that the value of 71 is an error in the data set and so could consider running their analyses both including and excluding this outlying value.

M6

Which one of the following statements is true?

a) One approach to handling outliers in a data set is to analyse the data both with and without the outliers and see whether the results are similar.

b) It is never sensible to transform data to overcome the problem of a skewed distribution as the parameter estimates obtained from the transformed data cannot be interpreted.

c) Outliers in data should be omitted from the analysis as they may skew the results.

d) An outlier is an extreme value which is incompatible with the main body of the data and is always greater than all the other values in the data set.

e) The only ways of dealing with outliers in a data set are to analyse the data both with and without the outliers and determine the effect of the omission, to omit the outlier(s) from the analysis or to transform the data.

M7

Consider the data relating to the number of eggs consumed in a week described in Questions M3 and M5. Which one of the following diagrams would be best for displaying the information?

a) A bar chart
b) A histogram
c) A pie chart
d) A scatter diagram
e) A segmented bar chart

M8

Consider the data on the number of eggs consumed in a week described in Questions M3 and M5. Which one of the following best describes the distribution of this variable?

a) Skewed to the right
b) Normally distributed
c) Skewed to the left
d) Uniformly distributed
e) Negatively skewed

M9

Which one of the following statements is true?

a) A pie chart is one in which a circular 'pie' is split into sectors, one for each category of a categorical variable, so that the area of each sector is equal.

b) A sensible way of displaying continuous numerical data is to draw a bar chart.

c) A histogram is a chart in which separate vertical (or horizontal) bars are drawn with gaps between the bars; the width (height) of each bar relates to a specific range of values of the variable, and its height (width) is proportional to the associated frequency of observations.

d) The distribution of a variable is right skewed if a histogram of observed values has a long tail to the right with one or a few high values.

e) A box-and-whisker plot comprises a vertical or horizontal rectangle indicating the interquartile range, within which is the median; the ends of the 'whiskers' represent the upper and lower limits of the 95% confidence interval for the median.

M10

The authors of the egg consumption study (Questions M3 and M5) now wish to summarise the data on the number of eggs consumed in a week. Which one of the following approaches would be the best way to summarise these data?

a) The arithmetic mean and range
b) The median and interquartile range
c) The median and range
d) The arithmetic mean and standard deviation
e) The mode

M11

Which one of the following statements is true?

a) The median is greater than the arithmetic mean if the data are skewed to the right.

b) The median value of n observations is equal to the $(n + 1)/2$th value in the ordered set if n is odd.

c) The median and the weighted mean are always identical if the weights used in the calculation of the weighted mean are equal.

d) The logarithmic transformation of left-skewed data will often produce a symmetrical distribution when the transformed data are plotted on an arithmetic scale.

e) The geometric mean of a data set is equal to the arithmetic mean of the log-transformed data.

M12

Study investigators collected information on haemoglobin levels in a sample of 212 healthy women of mixed ethnicity. The investigators calculated the median value, and used the 2.5th and 97.5th percentile values to generate a reference range. Which one of the following statements is true?

a) The authors generated the reference range using the percentile approach as the number of subjects in their study was small.

b) Healthy individuals in the population will not have a value of haemoglobin that falls below the lower limit of the reference range.

c) Use of the mean and standard deviation to generate the reference range would have provided a more suitable reference range.

d) Individuals in the population with an underlying health condition that has an impact on haemoglobin levels will always have values that fall outside the reference range.

e) An individual in the population with an underlying health condition that has an impact on haemoglobin levels is likely to have a value that falls outside the reference range.

M13

When numerical data are arranged in order of magnitude, which one of the following statements is true?

a) The interquartile range is the difference between the first and fourth percentiles.

b) The interdecile range contains the central 80% of the ordered observations.

c) The middle observation is always equal to the arithmetic mean.

d) The 50th percentile is equal to the fifth quartile.

e) The first percentile is always equal to the minimum value.

M14

If a set of observations follow the Normal or Gaussian distribution, which one of the following statements is true?

a) Its mean and variance are equal.

b) Its observations are derived from healthy individuals.

c) Its mean and variance are always equal to zero and one, respectively.

d) 95% of the observations lie between the mean ± 1.96 times the variance.
e) Approximately 68% of the observations lie between the mean ± the standard deviation.

M15

Which one of the following statements is true?
a) A Binomial random variable is the count of the number of events that occur randomly and independently in time or space at some fixed average rate.
b) The two parameters that characterise a Poisson distribution are the number of individuals in the sample (or repetitions of a trial) and the true probability of success for each individual (or in each trial).
c) The Chi-squared distribution is based on a categorical random variable.
d) When the logarithm of observations which follow the Lognormal distribution are taken, the transformed observations follow the Normal distribution.
e) The Lognormal distribution is highly skewed to the left.

M16

The distribution of age at menopause tends to be skewed to the left. Study investigators wish to identify demographic and socioeconomic factors that are independently associated with age at menopause. Which one of the following statements relating to the analysis of age at menopause is true?
a) The optimal analytical approach is always to use a nonparametric method due to the skewness of the distribution.
b) Use of the logarithmic transformation would permit a parametric analysis based on the Normal distribution.
c) Use of the square transformation may help to achieve Normality.
d) By using a square transformation, we can ensure that the assumptions underlying a parametric analysis based on the Normal distribution are met.
e) The study investigators would be best advised to categorise age at menopause before performing the analysis.

M17

Which one of the following statements is true?
a) The logistic transformation linearises a sigmoid curve.
b) The logistic transformation is generally applied to counts which follow the Poisson distribution.
c) If a numerical variable, y, is skewed to the right, the distribution of $z = y^2$ is often approximately Normal.
d) If a numerical variable, y, is skewed to the left, $z = \log y$ is often approximately Normally distributed.
e) The square transformation has properties which are similar to those of the logarithmic transformation.

Sampling and estimation

M18

Which one of the following statements is true? The sampling distribution of the mean:

a) represents the mean of the distribution obtained by taking many repeated samples of a fixed size from the population of interest and plotting the observations so obtained;
b) has a mean which is an unbiased estimate of the true mean in the population;
c) will follow a Normal distribution only if the distribution of the original data is Normal;
d) has a standard deviation which is larger than the standard error of the mean; or
e) cannot be drawn if the sample size of the repeated samples is small.

M19

Study investigators have collected data on the heights of a sample of 137 women in Thailand. Which one of the following statements is true?
a) The true mean height in the Thai female population will be equal to the mean height of the women in the sample.
b) If the investigators were to calculate the range of values determined by the mean height ± 1.96 × standard deviation, they would be able to assess from this range of values the precision of the estimated mean height in their sample.
c) To enable other research groups to compare the distribution of the height values in their own studies to those from the investigators' study, the investigators should calculate and present the median height and its associated confidence interval.
d) If the heights are approximately Normally distributed, the authors may calculate and present the mean height and its standard deviation. This will allow them to describe the distribution of height values in their sample.
e) By calculating the confidence interval for the mean, the investigators will be able to determine whether the height values in their sample are Normally distributed.

M20

Jensen *et al.* (2011) conducted a retrospective cohort study to assess the incidence of wound complications among patients undergoing lower-limb arthroplasty, before and after a change in clinical practice from the use of low-molecular-weight heparin to rivaroxaban. Prior to the switch to rivaroxaban, 9 of 489 patients (1.8%, 95% confidence interval 0.9 to 3.5%) returned to theatre with wound complications within 30 days compared to 22 of the 559 patients (3.9%, 95% confidence interval 2.6 to 5.9%) who received rivaroxaban. Which one of the following statements is true?
a) The confidence interval for the wound complication rate prior to the switch to rivaroxaban is asymmetrical, indicating that the outcome is not Normally distributed.
b) The true percentage of wound complications prior to the switch to rivaroxaban lies between 0.9% and 3.5%.
c) The 95% confidence intervals for the two periods overlap, indicating that there was no significant change in the wound complication rate after the switch to rivaroxaban.
d) Had the number of wound complications been greater in each period, the confidence intervals would have been wider.
e) Had the number of patients in each period been greater, the confidence intervals would have been narrower.

Jensen CD, Steval A, Partington PF, Reed MR, Muller SD. Return to theatre following total hip and knee replacement, before and after the introduction of rivaroxaban: a retrospective cohort study. J Bone Joint Surg Br 2011; 93: 91–5.

M21

Which of the following statements is true for a sample of size $n > 1$?

a) The 99% confidence interval for the mean is narrower than the 95% confidence interval for the mean.

b) The 95% confidence interval for the mean of a particular variable is narrower than the reference interval for that variable.

c) If the true standard deviation is known, the 95% confidence interval for the mean is calculated as the mean $\pm$ 1.96 times the standard deviation.

d) The 95% confidence interval for the mean represents the interval within which the sample mean falls with 95% certainty.

e) The 95% confidence interval for the mean represents the interval which contains the central 95% of the observations in the population.

Study design

M22

Which one of the following studies would be best described as a cohort study?

a) A study in which cells are stimulated with three different types of growth inducing protein.

b) A study of medical students who are followed from entering medical school to the end of their first year to describe the associations between lifestyle factors and end-of-first-year exam results.

c) A study of medical students who are split by the study investigators into two groups: those with surnames beginning with the letters A to M received regular counselling support over the first year, and those with surnames beginning with the letters O to Z did not. The outcome of the study was the proportion of students who passed their end-of-first-year exams, and this proportion was to be compared between the two groups.

d) Medical students who fail their end-of-first-year exams are interviewed about their lifestyles over the first year; a random sample of students who passed their end-of-first-year exams are also interviewed, and the results compared to assess the effects of lifestyle factors on failing the end-of-first-year exams.

e) Study investigators compared end-of-first-year exam pass rates at 10 different medical schools in the United Kingdom, and correlated these pass rates with the number of bars and nightclubs in the vicinity of each medical school.

M23

In medical research we are often interested in determining whether exposure to a factor causes an effect (e.g. a disease). Which one of the following criteria is a necessary component for assessing the cause of disease?

a) The cause and effect must take place simultaneously.

b) The association between cause and effect can be assessed on the basis of statistical results alone, independently of biological reasoning.

c) If feasible, removing the potential causative factor of interest should reduce the risk of disease.

d) The effect cannot be causal if the association between the cause and effect is small.

e) It is usually sufficient to imply causation on the basis of the results from a single study, provided the association between the cause and effect in that study is strong.

M24

Investigators conducted a randomised cross-over study to compare two appliances for the prevention of snoring. Every trial participant used each appliance for a period of one month, with a 2-week washout period between the two study periods. Which one of the following statements is true?

a) The investigators chose a cross-over design as the appliances are likely to have a long-term impact on snoring symptoms.

b) By using a cross-over design, the investigators were able to shorten the length of treatment time that was required.

c) Because they had used a cross-over design rather than a parallel group study design, the investigators had to increase the size of their sample.

d) A 2-week washout period was incorporated to allow the trial participants sufficient time to clean and return their appliances.

e) By choosing a cross-over design, the investigators were able to use each participant as his or her own control, thus reducing variability.

M25

In randomised trials of new human immunodeficiency virus therapies, investigators may use a composite endpoint known as the time to loss of virological response. Patients are deemed to meet the endpoint after the first of a series of events occurs: a new acquired immunodeficiency syndrome event, death, the patient is lost to follow-up or the patient experiences virological failure on treatment. At that point, the patient exits the trial and follow-up ceases on the patient. Which one of the following statements is true?

a) Investigators use a composite endpoint as they cannot make a decision in advance about which is the most important outcome.

b) Composite endpoints simplify the analysis of randomised trials.

c) If one or more components of the composite endpoint are deemed to have greater clinical relevance than others, then appropriate analytical methods which take this into consideration must be used when analysing a trial that utilises a composite endpoint.

d) A study that uses such a composite endpoint can provide reliable information about the frequency of occurrence of each component of the composite; thus, this type of trial provides good value for money.

e) If a composite endpoint is used instead of basing the analysis on each component of the composite, the length of the trial must be increased.

M26

Which one of the following statements is true?

a) A factorial design is one in which there is a single factor of interest.

b) A statistical interaction exists in a clinical trial when one or more of the treatments produce side effects.

c) The cross-over trial in a clinical setting is an example of a between-individual comparison.

d) A parallel trial comparing two treatments is one in which each individual receives both treatments in parallel.

e) A complete randomised design is one in which the experimental units are assigned randomly to the treatments and there are no other refinements to the design.

M27

Study investigators wish to perform a cluster randomised trial to evaluate the effectiveness of an education programme aimed at the parents of primary school children to increase the appropriate use, for this age group, of child restraints in cars. In the context of this study, 'parents' refers to the mother and/or father of a child, as appropriate. Rather than recruiting individual parents to the trial, the trial plans to recruit 32 primary schools with the intervention being applied at the school level (via meetings of groups of parents of children attending that school) – each school will be randomly assigned to receive the intervention or not. Which one of the following statements is true?

a) A cluster randomised design was chosen to reduce the size of the trial.

b) A cluster randomised design was chosen as it was possible to individually randomise the parents of each child to the intervention.

c) A cluster randomised design was chosen as it was felt that it would be impossible to treat the parents of each child in a school as an independent unit of investigation in the trial.

d) The unit of investigation for the trial is the individual adult driving each car.

e) The sample size for this trial is the same as it would have been had the investigators made the decision to use a nonclustered design.

M28

Which one of the following statements is true about clinical trials?

a) If a trial has secondary endpoints, there are two endpoints that are of primary interest.

b) Randomisation of individuals to patients is a process devised to avoid assessment bias.

c) A sequential trial is an extension of a cross-over trial when there are more than two treatments to be compared and each patient receives the treatments sequentially.

d) Blocked randomisation is used so as to achieve approximately equally sized groups at the end of patient recruitment.

e) Systematic allocation is a method of allocating individuals to treatments using a list of random numbers that has been created in a systematic way.

M29

Study investigators initiated a cohort study to determine the association between retirement and the incidence of depression within 5 years of retirement. The investigators recruited 1000 participants who were at the point of retirement; participants were then followed over a 5-year period with annual questionnaires sent to them to obtain information on self-reported depressive symptoms. Which one of the following statements is true?

a) By setting up a cohort in this way, the study investigators will be able to quantify the effect of retirement on the incidence of depression in the population within 5 years of retirement.

b) The investigators should restrict their analyses to the subgroup of participants who remain under follow-up for the full 5-year period.

c) The primary outcome measure of this study will be the prevalence of depression at 5 years.

d) To ensure that retirement precedes any symptoms of depression, the study investigators should exclude from their calculations of the incidence of depression any individual who already has depressive symptoms at recruitment.

e) This study is prone to recall bias as the information on depressive symptoms is obtained via self-report.

M30

Which one of the following statements is true about a cohort study?

a) The time sequence of events cannot be assessed.

b) It can provide information on a wide range of disease outcomes.

c) It is difficult to study exposure to factors that are rare.

d) The risk of disease cannot be measured directly.

e) It is generally cheap to perform.

M31

Kik *et al.* (2011) conducted an unmatched case–control study to investigate the extent to which travel to tuberculosis (TB)-endemic countries contributes to TB incidence among immigrants from Morocco living in the Netherlands. Cases were those of Moroccan background who had been diagnosed with TB in 2006–7 and had been seen at one of 17 municipal health services in the Netherlands; controls were a retrospective sample from the Survey on Integration of Minorities 2006 who did not have TB, had also been born in Morocco and were living in the Netherlands. Of the 32 cases with TB, 26 (81%) had travelled in the preceding year compared to 472 (58%) of the 816 controls. Which one of the following statements is true?

a) The risk of TB among Moroccan immigrants in the Netherlands is 32/816 (3.9%).

b) The risk of TB among Moroccan immigrants in the Netherlands is 32/848 (3.7%).

c) The odds ratio of TB is 1.40 (i.e. 81/58), suggesting that Moroccan immigrants in the Netherlands who travel to TB-endemic countries are 40% more likely to experience TB than those who do not travel to the TB-endemic countries.

d) The authors would be advised to report the relative risk from their study, as this would more accurately capture the increased risk of TB in Moroccan immigrants in the Netherlands associated with travel to TB-endemic countries than the odds ratio.

e) The odds ratio of TB is 3.16, suggesting that Moroccan immigrants in the Netherlands who travel to TB-endemic countries are over three times more likely to experience TB than those who do not travel to TB-endemic countries.

Kik SV, Mensen M, Beltman M, et al. *Risk of travelling to the country of origin for tuberculosis among immigrants living in a low-incidence country. Int J Tuberc Lung Dis 2011; 15: 38–43.*

M32

Which one of the following statements is true about a case–control study?

a) It is particularly suitable for rare diseases.

b) Loss to follow-up is a common problem.

c) The relative risk is commonly used to estimate the effect of the exposure on the disease outcome.

d) It is an example of a prospective observational study.

e) It is an example of an experimental study because those with disease are compared to those without it.

M33

In a recent matched case–control study, 200 cases with hepatocellular carcinoma were individually matched to 200 controls without hepatocellular carcinoma by sex and age (±5 years). The investigators collected information, for each subject, on a number of potential risk factors and were interested in determining which of them was associated with hepatocellular carcinoma. Which one of the following statements is true?

a) The authors should use conditional logistic regression methods to analyse the outcomes from this study.

b) The study investigators decided to match cases and controls by age and sex as they were particularly interested in the associations between each of these variables and hepatocellular carcinoma.

c) When calculating the odds ratios, the study investigators should ignore the fact that the cases and controls are matched by age and sex.

d) Had the authors loosened their matching criteria to ensure that cases and controls were matched by age within 10 rather than 5 years, the results from the study would have been strengthened.

e) The authors should use multiple linear regression methods to analyse the outcomes from this study.

Hypothesis testing

M34

Which one of the following statements is true?

a) If the hypothesised value for the effect of interest (e.g. the difference in means) in a hypothesis test lies within the 95% confidence interval for the effect, then we have evidence to reject the hypothesis, $P < 0.05$.

b) A hypothesis test of superiority which proceeds by calculating a test statistic and relating it to the appropriate probability distribution to obtain the P-value is so called because is it superior to testing the hypothesis using the relevant confidence interval.

c) The test statistic that is calculated in a hypothesis testing procedure reflects the amount of evidence in the data against the null hypothesis.

d) A bioequivalence trial is a particular type of randomised trial which is concerned with demonstrating that biological treatments have the same effect as nonbiological treatments on a disease outcome.

e) Nonparametric tests lead to an appreciation of the data, rather than focusing on decisions, because they do not concentrate on the parameters of the underlying distributions.

M35

Ogawa *et al.* (2010) conducted a study of 21 elderly women who participated in 12 weeks of resistance exercise training. The investigators measured muscle thickness and circulating levels of C-reactive protein, serum amyloid A, heat shock protein 70, tumour necrosis factor-α, interleukin-1, interleukin-6, monocyte chemotactic protein, insulin, insulin-like growth factor and vascular endothelial growth factor before and after the 12 weeks of training. Whilst training significantly reduced levels of five of the variables listed ($P < 0.05$), these reductions were not statistically significant after applying the Bonferroni correction. Which one of the following statements is true?

a) The authors used a Bonferroni correction to adjust their P-values as they did not believe that their initial findings were true.

b) The authors used a Bonferroni correction to adjust their P-values as they were performing subgroup analyses on the data set.

c) The authors used a Bonferroni correction to adjust their P-values as they were making multiple comparisons for a single outcome variable.

d) The authors used a Bonferroni correction to adjust their P-values and then applied a more stringent threshold than the conventional 0.05 for statistical significance.

e) The authors used a Bonferroni correction to adjust their P-values as they had multiple outcome variables.

Ogawa K, Sanada K, Machida S, Okutsu M, Suzuki K. Resistance exercise training-induced muscle hypertrophy was associated with reduction of inflammatory markers in elderly women. Mediators Inflamm 2010; 2010: 171023.

M36

Which one of the following statements is true about the probability of making a Type I error when performing a single hypothesis test?

a) It is equal to one minus the probability of a Type II error.

b) It is the probability of rejecting the null hypothesis when it is true.

c) It is the probability of not rejecting the null hypothesis when it is false.

d) It can never exceed 0.05.

e) It is equal to the significance level of the hypothesis test.

Basic techniques for analysing data

Numerical data

M37

McCorkle *et al.* (2010) measured spleen length in 66 tall athletes (defined as being at least 6 feet 2 inches tall for men and 5 feet 7 inches tall for women). Measurements of spleen size, obtained from an ultrasound examination, were compared to values from normal-sized individuals (not necessarily athletes) from the same population obtained from the published literature. The authors calculated the mean, standard deviation and variance of spleen length from their sample, and then conducted a one-sample *t*-test to determine whether the spleen length of tall athletes differed from that of the normal-sized individuals. Tall athletes had a mean spleen length of 12.19 cm (95% confidence interval 11.84, 12.55 cm), whereas the population mean spleen length was 8.94cm. Which one of the following statements is true?

a) The investigators chose to perform a one-sample t-test as they believed that the distribution of spleen length in the population was skewed.

b) The investigators chose to perform a one-sample t-test as their study included both male and female athletes.

c) From the information provided, it is likely that measurements of spleen length are highly skewed in the population.

d) As the authors included both male and female athletes of different sizes, the conclusions of the study must be unreliable.

e) The result of the one-sample t-test is statistically significant ($P < 0.05$) indicating that the mean spleen length of tall athletes was significantly greater than that of normal-sized individuals in the population.

McCorkle R, Thomas B, Suffaletto H, Jehle D. Normative spleen size in tall healthy athletes: implications for safe return to contact sports after infectious mononucleosis. Clin J Sport Med 2010; 20: 413–5.

M38

Which one of the following statements is true?

a) The one-sample t-test is used to test the null hypothesis that the sample mean takes a particular value.

b) The assumption underlying the one-sample t-test for small samples is that the variable of interest follows the t-distribution with degrees of freedom equal to the sample size minus one.

c) The sign test used on numerical data tests the null hypothesis that the population median takes a particular value.

d) The sign test used on numerical data evaluates the number of values in the sample that are greater (or less) than the median value specified in the null hypothesis and assesses whether it differs significantly from $n'/2$, where n' is the number of observations in the sample not equal to the specified median.

e) The sign test and one-sample t-test performed on the same set of numerical data will give exactly the same P-value if the data are Normally distributed.

M39

To investigate the value of information provided to patients at discharge following open-heart surgery, Ozcan *et al.* (2010) recruited 50 patients who underwent open-heart surgery from January to June 2007. At the time of discharge, all patients completed a pre-test questionnaire consisting of 34 questions that assessed their degree of knowledge relating to preventing re-hospitalisation, increasing self-care ability, gaining self-sufficiency and preventing complications post-surgery. Patients then underwent a training session and were provided with a booklet to take away with them. When patients attended for their routine medical follow-up after a one-month period, they completed the same questionnaire. The mean number of correct answers pre-intervention was 0.86 (standard deviation 1.28); this increased to 27.88 (3.84) after the intervention. Results of a Wilcoxon signed-ranks test suggested that the difference between the number of correct answers pre- and post-intervention was statistically significant ($P < 0.05$). Which one of the following statements is true?

a) It would have been preferable to use a two-sample t-test to analyse these data.

b) To gain a better understanding of the effect of the intervention, it would have been preferable to quote the median or mean change over time in the number of correctly answered questions (and the range or standard deviation of this, as appropriate), rather than the mean (standard deviation) number of correctly answered questions at each time point.

c) The Wilcoxon signed-ranks test is ideally suited to the situation where there are two independent data sets.

d) The result of the Wilcoxon signed-ranks test suggests that the apparent improvement in knowledge is likely to be a chance finding.

e) As there was a significant increase in knowledge level over the one-month period, the authors can conclude that their intervention was successful.

Ozcan H, Findik UY, Sut N. Information level of patients in discharge training given by nurses following open heart surgery. Int J Nurs Pract 2010; 16: 289–94.

M40

Which one of the following statements is true?

a) The sign test cannot be used on numerical data.

b) The Wilcoxon signed-ranks test is a more powerful test than the sign test when there are paired numerical observations.

c) The paired t-test is a nonparametric alternative to the Wilcoxon signed-ranks test.

d) The two-sample t-test produces the same P-value as the paired t-test when there are two groups of paired numerical observations.

e) The assumption underlying the paired t-test is that the variance of the observations is the same in each of the two groups.

M41

As part of a cross-sectional study to investigate risk factors for postpartum depression during the first postpartum year in women of low socioeconomic status, Yagmur and Ulukoca (2010) interviewed 785 women from Malatya in eastern Turkey. Data on depression were collected using the Edinburgh Postnatal Depression Scale (EPDS) which provides a value on a scale from 0 to 30 (higher scores indicate greater psychological distress), and through the Multidimensional Scale of Perceived Social Support (MSPSS) which provides a score that can range from 12 to 84 (higher scores indicate greater social support). Data were analysed using t-tests, one-way analysis of variance and logistic regression. Which one of the following statements is true?

a) Provided the assumptions of Normality and constant variance were satisfied, it would be appropriate to perform an unpaired t-test to investigate a possible association between the EPDS score and age group (categorised as ≤ 20, 21–30 and ≥ 31 years).

b) Provided the assumptions of Normality and constant variance were satisfied, it would be appropriate to perform a one-way analysis of variance to investigate a possible association between the EPDS score and age group (categorised as ≤ 20, 21–30 and ≥ 31 years).

c) As the range of values of the MSPSS scale is greater than that of the EPDS, it would be appropriate to use analysis of variance to assess the association between the two scores.

d) The investigators considered whether there was a difference in mean EPDS scores between those women who received health insurance and those who did not. The null hypothesis for this comparison was that those who received health insurance have a lower mean EPDS score than those who did not receive health insurance.

e) As each woman had a value of both the EPDS and the MSPSS scores, it would be appropriate to use a paired *t*-test to investigate whether there was an association between the two scores.

Yagmur Y, Ulukoca N. Social support and postpartum depression in low-socioeconomic level postpartum women in eastern Turkey. Int J Pub Health 2010; 55: 5439–49.

M42

Which one of the following statements is true?

a) The Wilcoxon signed-ranks test is a nonparametric alternative to the unpaired *t*-test.

b) The Wilcoxon signed-ranks test produces the same *P*-value as the Mann–Whitney *U*-test when comparing two groups of independent observations.

c) The null hypothesis for the unpaired *t*-test comparing two group means is that the sample means are equal in the population.

d) When the sample sizes are reasonably large, the unpaired *t*-test is robust to a departure from the underlying assumption of equal variances in the two groups.

e) When the sample sizes are reasonably large, the unpaired *t*-test is fairly robust to a departure from the assumption of Normality in each of the two groups.

M43

Which one of the following statements about the one-way analysis of variance to compare three independent groups of numerical observations is true?

a) The null hypothesis is that the sample variances are all equal.

b) The null hypothesis is that the population variances are all equal.

c) If the null hypothesis is rejected, then it can be concluded that at least one mean differs significantly from the others.

d) If the null hypothesis is rejected, then it can be concluded that all the three means differ significantly.

e) The sample sizes must be equal in the three groups.

Categorical data

M44

Following the use of a new experimental treatment for individuals with high blood pressure, study investigators noted that a small percentage of treated patients (7/212, 3.3%) experienced a rare adverse event within the first 6 months after treatment was started. In the general population, 1.3% of similarly aged individuals would be expected to experience the event over a similar period of time. Which one of the following statements is true?

a) It would be appropriate to use Fisher's exact test to compare the percentage experiencing the event in their study with the percentage that would be expected in the general population.

b) It would be appropriate to use the signed-ranks test to investigate whether the percentage of patients experiencing the event is higher than would be expected based on the general population figure.

c) As the percentage experiencing the event in the general population is known, it would be appropriate to compare the percentage of individuals who experienced the event in the study with the known percentage in the general population using a test statistic which relies on the Normal approximation to the Binomial distribution.

d) It would be appropriate to use a Chi-squared test to compare the percentage experiencing the event in their study with the percentage experiencing the event in the general population.

e) As the percentage experiencing the event in the general population is known, it would be appropriate to use McNemar's test to compare the percentage of individuals who experienced the event in their study with the known percentage in the general population.

M45

Which one of the following statements is true? When testing the null hypothesis that a single proportion in the population is equal to ½:

a) the test statistic follows the *t*-distribution with degrees of freedom equal to the number of observations minus one;

b) a continuity correction should be applied to the test statistic if referring that test statistic to the Normal distribution to obtain a *P*-value;

c) if the 95% confidence interval for the true proportion includes zero, the proportion is significantly different from ½, $P < 0.05$;

d) the data should be Normally distributed; or

e) none of the above.

M46

Investigators conducted a randomised controlled trial of a new dietary supplement (in conjunction with a low-fat diet) compared to a low-fat diet alone. The primary endpoint for the trial was weight loss of at least 10 kg over a 6-month period. Of 317 participants randomised to the low-fat diet alone, 218 (68.8%) achieved the primary endpoint; in comparison, of 321 participants randomised to the dietary supplement, 256 (79.8%) achieved the primary endpoint. The study investigators performed a Chi-squared test to compare the percentages achieving the primary endpoint in the two groups ($P = 0.002$). Which one of the following statements is true?

a) To calculate the expected number of participants randomised to the dietary supplement with the primary endpoint, it is necessary to multiply 321 by 0.798.

b) To calculate the expected number of participants randomised to the low-fat diet alone with the primary endpoint, it is necessary to multiply 321 by 0.743.

c) The authors did not need to use a continuity correction for the Chi-squared test, as the number of participants in each arm of the trial was large.

d) To complement the results of the Chi-squared test, the investigators should present some estimate of the treatment effect, such as the estimated difference in percentages achieving the endpoint in the two groups, with its associated confidence interval.

e) The investigators should have used logistic regression to adjust for potential confounders before concluding that the dietary supplement is associated with a significantly greater rate of weight loss than a low-fat diet alone.

M47

Which one of the following statements, relevant to the comparison of the proportion of individuals with a particular feature in two independent groups, is true?

a) The underlying assumption of the Chi-squared test to compare the two proportions is that the observed frequency in each of the four cells of the relevant contingency table should be at least five.

b) The underlying assumption of the Chi-squared test to compare the two proportions is that the expected frequency in each of the four cells of the relevant contingency table should be less than five.

c) The expected frequency in a given cell of the contingency table is the frequency that would be expected in that cell if the true proportions differ.

d) The Chi-squared test statistic should not include a continuity correction because the data are not continuous.

e) The degrees of freedom for the Chi-squared test is one.

M48

Lee *et al.* (2006) conducted a prospective cohort study of manuscripts reporting original research submitted to three major biomedical journals from November 2003 to February 2004. The primary aim of the study was to identify factors that were predictive of acceptance for publication. Of the 1107 manuscripts identified by the authors, 68 (6%) were accepted in total; the numbers accepted out of the numbers submitted for the three journals considered were 20/345 (6%), 25/381 (7%) and 23/381 (6%). Which one of the following statements is true?

a) A single Chi-squared test based on a 2×2 contingency table could be used to formally test whether the percentages accepted differed between at least two of the three journals.

b) A continuity correction must be applied when performing a Chi-squared test to compare the three percentages.

c) Due to the relatively small number of accepted papers, Fisher's exact test would be preferable to a Chi-squared test for these data.

d) Prior to performing a Chi-squared test, the authors should combine the data from two of the journals, and should compare the percentages accepted for the combined journal group with that of the third journal.

e) A Chi-squared test based on a 3×2 contingency table could be used to formally test whether the percentages accepted differed between at least two of the three journals.

Lee KP, Boyd EA, Holroyd-Leduc JM, Bacchetti P, Bero LA. Predictors of publication: characteristics of submitted manuscripts associated with acceptance at major biomedical journals. MJA 2006; 184: 621–6.

M49

Which one of the following statements about using the Chi-squared test to investigate the association between two factors is true, if one factor has r categories, the other has c categories and each individual can be classified into one category of each factor?

a) Both factors must be ordinal categorical variables if the Chi-squared test is to be applied.

b) McNemar's test is preferred to the Chi-squared test if more than 20% of the expected frequencies in the associated contingency table are less than five.

c) A continuity correction must be applied to the Chi-squared test statistic because the data are categorical and the Chi-squared distribution relates to a numerical variable.

d) The Chi-squared test statistic has one degree of freedom provided at least 80% of the expected frequencies in the associated contingency table are greater than or equal to five.

e) The Chi-squared test statistic has degrees of freedom equal to the product of $r - 1$ and $c - 1$.

Regression and correlation

M50

The study of 785 women from Malatya, described in Question M41, used the EPDS (with higher scores indicating greater psychological distress) and the MSPSS scale (with higher scores indicating greater perceived social support) to evaluate the risk factors for postpartum depression during the first postpartum year in women of low socioeconomic status. The investigators noted that the estimated Pearson correlation coefficient between the MSPSS and EPDS scores was -0.36 ($P < 0.0001$). Which one of the following statements is true?

a) The use of the Pearson correlation coefficient suggests that the distributions of both scores were skewed.

b) The result suggests that there is a tendency for the level of psychological distress experienced by these women to increase as perceived social support increases.

c) The authors found a strong correlation between perceived social support and psychological distress.

d) As the correlation coefficient is relatively small, there is no evidence of a linear association between the two scores.

e) The correlation coefficient suggests that psychological distress tends to decrease as the level of perceived social support increases.

M51

Which one of the following statements about the estimated Pearson correlation coefficient, r, describing the association between two variables, x and y, is true?

a) $0 \le r \le 1$.

b) If $r = 1$, there is no linear relationship between x and y.

c) If $r = 0$, there is no relationship between x and y.

d) Interchanging x and y will not affect the value of r.

e) The absolute value of r tends to decrease as the range of values of x and y increases.

M52

Which one of the following assumptions underlying a linear regression analysis between an explanatory variable, x, and a response variable, y, is true?

a) The x variable can be measured without error.

b) The values of y are Normally distributed in the population.

c) The values of x are Normally distributed in the population.

d) For each value of y, there is a distribution of values of x in the population: this distribution is Normal.

e) The variability of the x values in the population is the same for all values of y.

M53

In a study of the thoracic aortas of 80 subjects aged 0–20 years (Jo *et al.* 2010), thoracic aortic length was related to subject height through the estimated equation:

$$\text{Thoracic aortic length (cm)} = 1.7 + 0.1 \times \text{height (cm)}$$

Which one of the following statements is true?
a) There was an inverse linear relationship between thoracic aortic length and height in this study.
b) The predicted height for a subject with a thoracic aortic length of 14 cm is 1.23 m.
c) The predicted thoracic aortic length for a subject with a height of 1.23 m is 14 cm.
d) It is estimated that, on average, thoracic aortic length is increased by 1 cm for each additional metre increase in height.
e) Prior to fitting the regression equation, the investigators could have re-scaled the height variable by multiplying it by 10, resulting in a more clinically relevant parameter estimate.

Jo CO, Lande MB, Meagher CC, Wang H, Vermilion RP. A simple method of measuring thoracic aortic pulse wave velocity in children: methods and normal values. J Am Soc Echocardiogra 2010; 23: 735–40.

M54

Which one of the following statements relating to a univariable linear regression analysis between a dependent variable, y, and an explanatory variable, x, is truc?
a) Goodness of fit of the regression line may be assessed by evaluating the Pearson correlation coefficient between the two variables: it represents the proportion of variability of y that can be explaincd by its linear relationship with x.
b) If a test of the hypothesis that the true intercept is zero is statistically significant ($P < 0.05$), this provides evidence that there is a linear relationship between the two variables.
c) We generally choose to centre the explanatory variable when the intercept of the model does not provide a predicted value of the dependent variable for a meaningful individual.
d) We generally choose to scale the explanatory variable when the intercept of the model does not provide a predicted value of the dependent variable for a meaningful individual.
e) An outlier is always an influential point.

M55

Based on anthropometric data from 212 study volunteers aged 13–27 years (Bouzgarou *et al.* 2011), it has been estimated that peak nasal inspiratory flow can be predicted by the following equation:

$$\text{Peak nasal inspiratory flow (l/min)} = 1.4256 \times \text{height (cm)}$$
$$+ 33.0215 \times \text{gender (where 0 = female and 1 = male)}$$
$$+ 1.4117 \times \text{age (years)} - 136.6778.$$

Which one of the following statements is true?
a) The intercept of the multiple regression model provides an estimate of the predicted peak nasal inspiratory flow for a typical male aged 13–27 years.
b) Predicted peak nasal inspiratory flow is lower in males than in females.

c) A good estimate of peak inspiratory flow for a female aged 55 years who is 1.63 m tall is 173.34 l/min.
d) If gender were to be categorised as 1 = female and 0 = male, the parameter estimate for gender would remain the same but its sign would have been reversed.
e) If gender were to be recategorised as 1 = female and 0 = male, the intercept would remain unchanged.

Bouzgarou MD, Saad HB, Chouchane A, Cheikh IB, Zbidi A, Dessanges JF, Tabka Z. North African reference equation for peak nasal inspiratory flow. J Laryngol Otol 2011; 125: 595–602.

M56

Which one of the following statements concerning a multivariable linear regression analysis is true?
a) If the computer output contains an analysis of variance table, the F-test will be testing the null hypothesis that all the partial regression coefficients are equal to zero.
b) A given partial regression coefficient represents the average change in the associated explanatory variable for a unit change in the dependent variable.
c) We can perform a multivariable linear regression analysis if the dependent variable is binary or numerical.
d) One of the reasons for performing the multivariable linear regression analysis is to determine the extent to which one or more of the explanatory variables is (or are) linearly related to the dependent variable, after adjusting for the other covariates that may be related to it.
e) Collinearity is present if the dependent variable and at least one of the explanatory variables are highly correlated.

M57

Nabi *et al.* (2006) used a self-administered questionnaire to collect data on sleepiness and other driving behaviours in members of the GAZEL cohort, a large cohort of men and women working at a French national electricity and gas company (GAZEL is an abbreviation of the words *gaz and electricité*). Of the 13 674 participants included in the study, 8597 (62.9%) reported that they had never driven while sleepy, 4917 (36%) reported that they had driven while sleepy a few times in the past year, 104 (0.8%) reported driving while sleepy about once a month, 35 (0.3%) about once a week and 21 (0.2%) more than once a week. The authors used logistic regression to identify factors associated with driving while sleepy. In unadjusted analyses, the odds ratio for driving while sleepy among respondents who reported having retired from work was 0.5 (95% confidence interval 0.5 to 0.6); after adjustment for many factors relating to lifestyle and working conditions, the odds ratio increased to 0.9 (0.8 to 1.4). Which one of the following statements is true?
a) Being retired has a significant independent protective effect against driving while sleepy.
b) Although it appears from univariable analyses that being retired is protective against driving while sleepy, it is more likely that this association can be explained by confounding with lifestyle factors and working conditions.
c) After controlling for possible confounders, there was an increased odds of driving while sleepy among those who were retired.

d) After controlling for lifestyle and working conditions, there was a reduction in the odds of driving while sleepy in those who were retired.

e) As the outcome variable was ordinal, it would have been preferable to have performed a multiple linear regression analysis.

Nabi H, Gueguen A, Chiron M, Lafont S, Zins M, Lagarde E. Awareness of driving while sleepy and road traffic accidents: prospective study in GAZEL cohort. BMJ 2006; 333(7558): 75.

M58

Which one of the following statements about linear logistic regression analysis is true?

a) In the logistic regression equation, the coefficient attached to a particular explanatory variable represents the odds of the outcome of interest (e.g. disease) when the variable takes the value $(x + 1)$ relative to the odds of disease when the variable takes the value x, whilst adjusting for all the other explanatory variables in the model.

b) Logistic regression analysis can be performed only if all of the explanatory variables are binary.

c) The model Chi-square (also called the Chi-square for covariates) tests the null hypothesis that all the regression coefficients in the model are zero.

d) The deviance (also called the LRS or −2log likelihood) tests the null hypothesis that all the regression coefficients in the model are zero.

e) One of the assumptions underlying the logistic regression analysis is that the dependent variable is Normally distributed for each value of each of the explanatory variables.

M59

In a study of pregnancy rates in 225 women living with HIV in Brazil (Friedman *et al.* 2011), 60 pregnancies occurred over a total follow-up period of 565 person-years. Which one of the following statements is true?

a) The pregnancy rate in this sample was 0.27 per person-year.

b) The pregnancy rate in this sample was 1.06 per person-year.

c) One pregnancy occurred in this sample every 0.94 person-years.

d) One pregnancy occurred in this sample every 9.4 person-years.

e) Based on the estimated rate in the sample, if each woman had been followed for 3 years, 180 pregnancies would have occurred.

Friedman RK, Bastos RI, Leite IC, et al. *Pregnancy rates and predictors in women with HIV/AIDS in Rio de Janeiro, southeastern Brazil. Rev Saude Publica 2011; 45: 373–81.*

M60

In 2002, new legislation was introduced in Alberta, Canada that mandated the wearing of bicycle helmets when cycling for those aged <18 years. Using data from two comparative studies conducted in Calgary and in Edmonton in 2000 (2 years prior to the new legislation) and in 2006 (4 years after the introduction of the legislation), Karkhaneh *et al.* (2011) described changes in helmet usage in children (<13 years), adolescents (13–17 years) and adults (≥18 years). To estimate the changes in helmet usage, the authors used Poisson regression models which included calendar year (2000 for the reference group or 2006 otherwise) as a covariate; the parameter estimate relating to calendar year from the model provides an estimate of the proportional change in helmet usage from 2000 to 2006. After controlling for city, location type (residential area, school, college, park, commuter route or designated cycling path), companion helmet use (riding alone, riding with at least one other helmeted person or riding with others, none of whom are helmeted), the proportion of individuals in the neighbourhood aged <18, socioeconomic status and weather conditions, the authors reported that helmet use increased by 29% in children (relative rate 1.29, 95% confidence interval 1.20 to 1.39), by 112% in adolescents (2.12, 95% confidence interval 1.75 to 2.56) and by 14% in adults (1.14, 95% confidence interval 1.02 to 1.27). Which one of the following statements is true?

a) To investigate whether the legislation had a greater impact in Edmonton than Calgary, a test for a statistical interaction between city and calendar year should be performed.

b) The authors adjusted for companionship, as children would rarely be expected to cycle alone.

c) The impact of the legislation on helmet wearing is significantly lower among adults than among children.

d) By controlling for city, the authors have allowed the impact of the legislation on helmet use to be different in Edmonton and Calgary.

e) To formally test whether the legislation had a greater impact on helmet wearing in Edmonton than in Calgary, the authors should stratify the data set by city, and perform the regression analysis separately for those in each city.

Karkhaneh M, Rowe BH, Saunders LD, Voaklander DC, Hagel BE. Bicycle helmet use four years after the introduction of helmet legislation in Alberta, Canada. Accid Anal Prev 2011; 43: 788–96.

M61

In a multivariable regression model to identify factors associated with an increased risk of myocardial infarction, the latest triglyceride level (measured in mmol/l) was included as a covariate after a $\log_2$ transformation. The estimated relative rate of myocardial infarction associated with the latest $\log_2$ triglyceride level from the Poisson regression model was 1.35. Which one of the following statements is true?

a) For every doubling in the latest triglyceride level, an individual's rate of experiencing a myocardial infarction was increased by 35%.

b) For every 1 mmol/l increment in the latest triglyceride level, an individual's rate of experiencing a myocardial infarction was increased by 35%.

c) Taking a logarithmic transformation of the latest triglyceride level is unlikely to have an impact on the P-value associated with the covariate in the model.

d) The assumed apparent association between the rate of myocardial infarction and the triglyceride level (mmol/l) in this model is log-linear.

e) If a $\log_{10}$ rather than a $\log_2$ transformation had been taken of the latest triglyceride level, the P-value associated with the covariate may have been different.

Table M62.1 Summary data for patients in observational study

	All patients	Receiving new drug	
		Yes	No
Number of patients	12261	895	11366
Male gender; n (%)	5303 (43.3)	473 (52.8)	4830 (42.5)
Median (interquartile range) age (years)	46 (33 to 57)	51 (35 to 64)	45 (32 to 57)
Current cigarette smoker; n (%)	4051 (33.0)	289 (32.2)	3762 (33.1)

M62

Male sex, current smoking and older age are three of the known risk factors for cardiovascular disease (CVD) in the general population. Using information collected as part of an observational study of 12261 individuals diagnosed with cancer, investigators considered whether the use of a new treatment for cancer was associated with an increased risk of CVD. Over a total follow-up of 41443 person-years, there were 247 episodes of CVD, of which 20 occurred in the 895 patients (2712 person-years) who received the new drug. Selected characteristics of the patients in the study (hypothetical data) are shown in Table M62.1. The crude estimate of the relative rate of CVD among those receiving the new drug compared to those not receiving the drug was 1.26. Which one of the following statements is true?
a) Adjusting the relative rate estimate for differences in gender is likely to lead to an increase in its value.
b) Adjusting the relative rate estimate for differences in age is likely to lead to a reduction in its value.
c) Current cigarette smoking is likely to be a strong confounder in this analysis.
d) The relative rate of 1.26 indicates that receipt of the new drug is independently associated with an increased rate of CVD.
e) After adjustment for age and gender, the relative rate estimate dropped to 1.10; thus, the new drug can be blamed for 10% of the CVD events that occurred.

M63

Which one of the following statements about Poisson regression is true?
a) It is appropriate to perform a Poisson regression analysis when interest is focussed on determining the relationship between a binary outcome variable and a number of explanatory variables which may be numerical and/or categorical and where all individuals are followed for the same length of time.
b) The exponential of a particular partial Poisson regression coefficient is interpreted as a relative rate associated with a unit increase in the relevant variable, after adjustment for all other covariates in the model.
c) The effects of the different covariates in the Poisson regression model are additive on the rate of disease (if disease is the outcome of interest).
d) Extra-Poisson variation occurs when the residual variance is less than would be expected from a Poisson model.
e) Variables that change over time cannot be incorporated in a Poisson regression model.

M64

Which one of the following statements about a generalised linear model (GLM) is true?
a) The method of least squares is used to estimate the regression coefficients in all GLMs.
b) The link function in a logistic GLM is often referred to as the identity link.
c) The likelihood is the probability of the model, given the data.
d) Maximum likelihood estimation of the coefficients of the GLM is an iterative process that maximises the likelihood.
e) The adequacy of fit of all GLMs is determined by evaluating the square of the correlation coefficient, representing the proportion of the variability of the outcome variable that can be explained by its relationship with the covariates in the model.

M65

Which one of the following statements about explanatory variables in statistical models is true?
a) It is necessary to create indicator or dummy variables for all categorical explanatory variables that have more than two categories.
b) Confounding between explanatory variables in the model is also called effect modification.
c. Effect modification occurs in a statistical model when two or more of the explanatory variables are highly correlated.
d) Using automatic selection procedures to identify the optimal model by selecting only some of the explanatory variables to be included in the final model is particularly useful when interest is focussed on gaining insight into whether an explanatory variable influences an outcome or in estimating its effect on the outcome.
e) A model is over-fitted when it includes an excessive number of explanatory variables.

Important considerations

M66

Which one of the following statements is true?
a) Selection bias in a clinical trial is likely to occur when randomisation is not used to determine to which treatments the subjects will be allocated.
b) Increasing the sample size will always reduce bias in a study.
c) The ecological fallacy results in a bias which sometimes occurs when we believe mistakenly that an association we observe between variables in individuals reflects the corresponding association at an aggregate level.
d) A confounding variable is an exposure variable that is related to both the outcome of interest (e.g. disease) and one (or more) of the other exposure variables.
e) A confounding variable is an outcome variable (e.g. disease) that is related to two (or more) exposure variables.

M67

Which one of the following statements is true?
a) The linearity assumption in a univariable linear regression analysis can be checked by performing Levene's test.

b) The linearity assumption in a univariable linear regression analysis is satisfied if the scatter of the points in a plot of the residuals against the explanatory variable is random.

c) The linearity assumption in a univariable linear regression analysis is satisfied if the scatter of points in a plot of the residuals against the explanatory variable exhibits a linear relationship.

d) A sensitivity analysis may be used to assess how sensitive the conclusions of a hypothesis test are to a change in significance level.

e) It is always sensible to analyse a data set in many different ways, by using multiple different statistical tests which essentially investigate the same or similar hypotheses, and then to display their results in order to show that any conclusions are robust to the method of analysis.

M68

Investigators are designing a randomised controlled trial of a new drug for the treatment of hypertension. Patients will be randomised, in a 1:1 ratio, to receive either standard-of-care or the new drug. The authors believe that 70% of patients receiving standard-of-care will reach the primary endpoint for the trial after 1 year. They have set the power of the trial at 80% and will use an alpha (significance level) of 5%. The minimum clinically relevant treatment effect is assumed to be 10%. Using these specifications, they estimate that they will have to recruit 626 patients to the trial, 313 in each arm. Assuming that all other factors which affect sample size estimation remain constant, other than that specified in the statement, which one of the following statements is true?

a) If the investigators reduce the power to 70%, they would have to increase the numbers required for their trial.

b) If the investigators reduce alpha to 1%, they would have to decrease the numbers required for their trial.

c) If the investigators increase the power to 90%, they would have to increase the numbers required for their trial.

d) The investigators now believe that their initial estimate, that 70% of patients on standard-of-care will reach the primary endpoint, is too high and wish to reduce this to 60%; accordingly, they will have to decrease the numbers required for the trial.

e) Changing the minimum clinically relevant treatment effect to 15% will have no impact on the numbers required for the trial.

M69

Which one of the following statements is true?

a) Fagan's nomogram is useful for sample size determination.

b) If it is necessary to conduct a pilot study for sample size estimation, the pilot study data should never be incorporated into the main study database.

c) A power statement indicates that the statistical methods used are robust.

d) The optimal sample size of a study can be reduced if the significance level of the proposed test is lowered from 0.05 to 0.01.

e) If it is decided that the power of the study should be raised from 80% to 90%, the sample size should be increased to accommodate this.

M70

Which one of the following statements is true?

a) The CONSORT Statement provides a useful set of guidelines for reporting the results of a randomised controlled trial.

b) The STROBE Statement provides a useful set of guidelines for reporting the results of a meta-analysis.

c) The QUORUM Statement provides a useful set of guidelines for reporting the results when there are only a small number of individuals involved in the study.

d) The EQUATOR Network was initiated with the objective of providing resources and training for the reporting of health research in developing countries around the equator.

e) It is not necessary to report in a publication which computer package was used to analyse the data in the study unless the data are made available to those reading the publication.

Additional techniques

M71

Urinalysis provides a relatively costly but accurate test for proteinuria (i.e. when the albumin–creatinine ratio (ACR) is greater than or equal to 30 mg/g). White *et al.* (2011) investigated the ability of a cheaper urine dipstick test to identify those with proteinuria. Based on data from 10 944 individuals with complete urinalysis data, White *et al.* investigated the ability of an ACR value $\geq$30 mg/g measured on a urine dipstick to identify individuals with ACR $\geq$30 mg/g based on urinalysis. The area under the receiver operating characteristic curve (AUROC) for dipstick detection of ACR $\geq$30 mg/g was 0.85 in men and 0.78 in women. Which one of the following statements is true?

a) Among men, an ACR of $\geq$30 mg/g from a urine dipstick will correctly identify 85% of those who really do have proteinuria.

b) The AUROC of 0.78 in women indicates that 78% of those with a raised ACR on a dipstick will truly have proteinuria based on urinalysis.

c) The AUROC is calculated as sensitivity divided by (1 minus specificity).

d) Given two randomly selected women from the sample, one of whom does and one of whom does not have ACR $\geq$30 mg/g based on dipstick analysis, the woman with the ACR $\geq$30 mg/g based on dipstick analysis has a 78% probability of also having an ACR $\geq$30 mg/g based on urinalysis.

e) Given two randomly selected women from the sample, one of whom does and one of whom does not have proteinuria based on urinalysis, the dipstick analysis will correctly identify the woman with proteinuria on 78% of occasions.

White SL, Yu R, Craig JC, Polkinghorne KR, Atkins RC, Chadban SJ. Diagnostic accuracy of urine dipsticks for detection of albuminuria in the general community. Am J Kidney Dis 2011; 58: 19–28.

M72

Which one of the following statements about a diagnostic test is true?

a) The sensitivity of the test is equal to the proportion of individuals without the disease who are correctly identified by the test.

b) The specificity of the test is equal to the proportion of individuals with the disease who are correctly identified by the test.

c) The positive predictive value of the test is the proportion of individuals with a positive test result who have the disease.

d) The positive predictive value of the test is the proportion of individuals with the disease who are correctly identified by the test.

e) The likelihood ratio for a positive test result is the chance that the patient has the disease if he or she tests positive for it divided by the chance that the patient has the disease if he or she tests negative.

M73

Quint *et al.* (2011) compared two different laboratory assays to distinguish between lymphogranuloma venereum (LGV) and non-LGV *Chlamydia trachomatis* infections (the latter being further subcategorised as non-LGV, non-LGV+LGV and untypable). A total of 201 positive rectal swabs were available for analysis, of which 99 had previously been diagnosed as LGV using algorithm 1 (Aptima Combo 2 assay followed by an in-house *pmpH* LGV polymerase chain reaction (PCR)). The authors retested all 201 samples using a second algorithm (genoTyping Reverse Hybridization Assay, or Ct-DT RHA) and calculated Cohen's kappa for four categories; the estimated kappa value was 0.90 with 94% of samples showing diagnostic concordance. Which one of the following statements is true?

a) The kappa coefficient was calculated as the authors wished to assess the repeatability of algorithm 1.

b) Had the authors combined some of the non-LGV subcategories before calculating kappa, the kappa value would probably have decreased.

c) To formally test whether the two algorithms agree, a significance test of the null hypothesis that the true value of kappa equals 0 should be conducted.

d) According to the classification by Landis and Koch (1977), the value of the kappa coefficient indicates that there was substantial agreement between the two algorithms.

e) The kappa coefficient was calculated as the authors wished to assess method agreement between the two algorithms.

Quint KD, Bom RJM, Quint WGV, Bruisten SM et al. Anal infections with concomitant Chlamydia trachomatis *genotypes among men who have sex with men in Amsterdam, the Netherlands. BMC Infect Dis 2011; 11: 63.*
Landis JR and Koch GG. The measurement of observer agreement for categorical data. Biometrics 1977; 33: 159–74.

M74

Which one of the following statements about measuring the agreement between pairs of observations is true?

a) Cohen's kappa is used to measure the agreement when the responses are categorical, and is equal to the proportion of pairs that agree.

b) We can calculate a weighted kappa value to measure the agreement when the data are measured on a nominal categorical scale and there are more than two categories of response.

c) The intra-class correlation coefficient is an index of agreement which takes values from −1 to +1.

d) The Pearson correlation coefficient is an appropriate measure of agreement when the responses are measured on a numerical scale.

e) If the data are measured on a numerical scale and the difference between each pair of responses is determined and their distribution is approximately Normal, the limits of agreement in a Bland and Altman diagram indicate the range of values within which 95% of the differences are expected to lie.

M75

Which one of the following statements about evidence-based medicine is true?

a) The hierarchy of evidence indicates that a randomised controlled trial always provides stronger evidence than a cohort study.

b) Published papers always provide all the relevant information (e.g. on diagnosis, prognosis or therapy) required for an evidence-based investigation.

c) Using evidence-based medicine means that a novel therapy will not be adopted in the community unless a relevant randomised controlled trial shows a statistically significant effect when compared to a control therapy.

d) The number needed to treat (or harm) expresses the effectiveness (or safety) of an intervention in a way that is clinically meaningful.

e) An evidence-based approach is restricted to conventional therapeutic interventions and can never be applied to alternative medicine.

M76

Study investigators were interested in the association between infections that are common in childhood and longer term clinical outcomes. To study this, they recruited children aged 5–8 years living in three cities in the United Kingdom (Liverpool, London and Bath). Within each city, three primary schools were selected and all the children in one class (selected at random) in every school were invited to participate. The children were followed over a one-year period during which time all infections that occurred were recorded. The children were then re-contacted 10 years later, at which stage any clinical conditions that had occurred over the past 10 years were recorded. Which one of the following statements is true?

a) The data collected conform to a two-level nested structure.

b) The children's class is the level 1 unit for the analysis.

c) The city in which the children live is the level 4 unit for the analysis.

d) The data collected conform to a three-level nested structure.

e) As the class in each school was selected randomly, there is no need for the authors to take account of the class in the analysis.

M77

Consider the situation when 60 patients have been assigned randomly to one of two treatments, A or B, and every patient has an observation at each of six successive time points. Interest is centred on comparing A and B. Which one of the following statements is true?

a) When analysing the data, failure to take account of the lack of independence between the repeated observations in each patient usually results in overestimation of the standard errors of the estimates of interest.

b) A simple appropriate way of analysing such data is to base the analysis for each patient on a single summary measure that captures important aspects of the data.

c) A simple appropriate way of analysing such data is to compare the mean responses at each time point separately using an unpaired *t*-test.

d) A simple appropriate way of analysing such data is to perform a one-way analysis of variance comparing the means in the two groups at each of the different time points.

e) If a linear relationship between the response and time is appropriate, a simple and sensible way of analysing the data is to fit a single linear regression line to the data for all the patients in a treatment group and then compare the slopes of the two lines (one for A and one for B) so obtained.

M78

Which one of the following statements concerning a regression analysis of a two-level structure of individual units within a cluster (e.g. teeth within a patient's mouth) is true?

a) If the clustering is ignored, spuriously significant results may be obtained.

b) A random effects model is not appropriate for the analysis of the data unless randomisation has been used at the design stage of the study.

c) If a random effects model were used to analyse the data, it would differ from the model which takes no account of the clustering because the latter does not incorporate random error into it.

d) Random effects models are also known as population-averaged or marginal models.

e) The intra-class correlation coefficient expresses the variation between the individual units within a cluster as a proportion of the total variation.

M79

Rahimi *et al.* (2011) conducted a meta-analysis of published and unpublished findings from large statin trials with the aim of investigating whether long-term treatment with statins can reduce the risk of atrial fibrillation. Twenty-nine trials were included in the analysis, although the primary analysis was restricted to 22 trials that compared a statin with a control regimen; in these trials, the overall odds ratio for atrial fibrillation in those receiving statins compared to those receiving a control was 0.95 (95% confidence interval 0.88 to 1.03). A test for heterogeneity gave a Chi-squared value of 21.9 (21 degrees of freedom, $P = 0.40$). Which one of the following statements is true?

a) The test for heterogeneity suggests that the combined estimate of the odds ratio from the meta-analysis should be interpreted with caution.

b) There is no evidence from the meta-analysis that statin treatment has a genuine effect on the odds of atrial fibrillation.

c) The authors should have calculated the combined estimate of the odds ratio using a random effects meta-analysis.

d) Statins were shown to significantly reduce the odds of atrial fibrillation in this meta-analysis.

e) The authors presented a forest plot – this allowed them to investigate whether the results of their study were likely to have been affected by publication bias.

Rahimi K, Martin J, Emberson J, McGale P, Majoni W, Merhi A, Asselbergs FW, Krane V, Macfarlane PW. Effects of statins on atrial fibrillation: collaborative meta-analysis of published and unpublished evidence from randomised controlled trials. BMJ 2011; 342: d1250 (online).

M80

Which one of the following statements about a meta-analysis is true?

a) A component of evidence-based medicine is a meta-analysis which focuses on systematic reviews of large studies.

b) The hypothesis test of homogeneity in a meta-analysis tests the null hypothesis that there is no clinical variation between the included studies.

c) A random effects meta-analysis is often used instead of a fixed effects meta-analysis if there is evidence of statistical heterogeneity.

d) The index, I^2, used to quantify the impact of heterogeneity in a meta-analysis depends on the number of studies included in the meta-analysis.

e) Publication bias in a meta-analysis may be elicited by drawing a forest plot and noting whether the shape of the points is skewed or asymmetrical.

M81

The Cancer Prevention Study II (Harris *et al.* 2004) followed a cohort of 364 239 men and 576 535 women for a period of 6 years to determine rates of death from cancer of the trachea, bronchus or lung. The authors considered the association between mortality rates and the tar level of the cigarettes smoked by the subset of men in the study who were current smokers in 1982. Compared to men who smoked cigarettes with a tar content of 15–21 mg, the mortality hazard ratios among those who smoked cigarettes with a tar content of 0–7 mg, 8–14 mg and ≥ 22 mg were 1.17 (95% confidence interval 0.95 to 1.45), 1.02 (0.90 to 1.16) and 1.44 (1.20 to 1.73), respectively. Which one of the following statements is true?

a) There is no evidence from this study that the tar content of the cigarettes smoked is associated with an increased mortality rate from cancer of the trachea, bronchus or lung.

b) Men who smoked cigarettes with a tar content of ≥ 22 mg had a significantly increased risk of mortality from cancer of the trachea, bronchus or lung compared to men who smoked cigarettes with a tar content of 0–7 mg.

c) The authors would have been able to more usefully estimate the association between tar content and mortality risk if they had included tar content as a continuous covariate in their analysis.

d) The reference group for the analysis was men who did not smoke cigarettes in 1982.

e) Had the authors changed the reference group for the analysis to men who smoked cigarettes with a tar content of ≥ 22 mg, the relative hazard estimate for those smoking cigarettes with a tar content of 15–21 mg would have been less than 1.

Harris JE, Thun MJ, Mondul AM, Calle EE. Cigarette tar yields in relation to mortality from lung cancer in the Cancer Prevention Study II prospective cohort, 1982–8. BMJ 2004; 328: 72.

M82

Which one of the following statements about survival analysis is true?

a) What is of primary importance in a survival analysis is whether or not the individual reaches the endpoint (e.g. death).

b) Survival times are right-censored where follow-up does not begin until after the baseline date.

c) Informative censoring means that full information is available on why and when an individual's follow-up is censored.

d) The relative hazard is assumed to be constant in a Cox proportional hazards model.

e) The log-rank test in a Kaplan–Meier survival analysis is a parametric test, comparing the survival experience in two or more groups, which assumes that the logarithm of the ranked data are Normally distributed.

M83

Which one of the following statements is true?

a) The Bayesian approach to inference tends to over-emphasise the role of hypothesis testing and whether or not a result is statistically significant.

b) One of the disadvantages of a Bayesian analysis is the subjective nature of the prior so that its specification is often criticised as arbitrary.

c) Altman's nomogram is a diagram which can be used to interpret a diagnostic test result using a Bayesian approach.

d) In the context of a diagnostic test, Bayes theorem converts the observed test result into the probability that the individual does or does not have the disease.

e) In the context of a diagnostic test, the likelihood of a positive test result describes the probability that the individual has the disease if he or she tests positive for it.

M84

Study investigators wished to generate a new prognostic score that could identify patients at high risk of mortality during intensive care unit (ICU) admission. To generate the score, the investigators captured data on 25 variables from 236 individuals admitted to an ICU at a single hospital between 1 January and 31 December 2008; the outcome of the study was death during the current ICU admission. Based on the data collected, they generated a score for predicting the risk of ICU mortality. The AUROC for this score was 0.756, and the Hosmer–Lemeshow goodness of fit statistic gave a P-value of 0.06. The investigators then applied the score to the next 50 admissions at their ICU; the AUROC for this validation data set was 0.712. On the basis of these findings, the investigators recommended that other units should start to use this score routinely to identify patients at high risk of mortality during ICU admission. Which one of the following statements is true?

a) The investigators retested their score on a validation sample because the estimate of the AUROC from the sample on which the score was based was likely to have been overly optimistic.

b) The investigators have provided strong evidence that the model is well calibrated.

c) By applying their model to another set of patients, the investigators have provided strong evidence that their model is transportable.

d) Had the investigators used cross-validation on their sample, they would have been able to demonstrate that the score had been externally validated.

e) The AUROC value for the validation sample suggests that this prognostic score may be no better than chance at identifying patients who are likely to die during ICU admission.

M85

Which one of the following statements about a prognostic score is true?

a) A prognostic score describes the probability that an individual falls into one particular category of an exposure variable.

b) A receiver operating characteristic curve is used to assess the extent to which the prognostic score is correctly calibrated.

c) Bootstrapping is an internal validation procedure which can be used to estimate the prognostic score and assess its performance.

d) The Hosmer–Lemeshow goodness of fit statistic can be used to provide a graded measure of the likelihood that an individual will experience the event of interest.

e) A regression model is always used to generate a prognostic score.

Part 2: Structured Questions

S1

Table S1.1 shows a portion of a data set (stored in Excel) that was created to collect data for a study on risk factors for myocardial infarction (MI), the primary outcome of the study. Eligible individuals who had not previously experienced any cardiovascular disease (including MI) were recruited from January to December 2000 and were males and females aged 30–65 years. Information was collected on a total of 1113 individuals; only data for the first 30 individuals are shown in Table S1.1. The variables collected were:

Study ID:	Unique study identifier
Entry date:	Date of recruitment in study
Sex:	M = Male, F = Female
Age:	Age (years)
Ethnic group:	1 = White; 2 = Black African; 3 = Other black; 4 = Other; 9 = Not known
Smoking:	0 = Never smoker; 1 = Current smoker; 2 = Ex-smoker; 9 = Unknown
BMI:	Body mass index (kg/m^2)
TC:	Total cholesterol (mmol/L)
HDL-C:	High-density lipoprotein cholesterol (mmol/L)
TG:	Triglyceride (mmol/L)
LLD:	Any receipt of lipid-lowering drugs (y = yes, n = no)
Date of first MI:	Date of first MI during study.

Overall, a total of 25 patients experienced an MI over a total follow-up period of 6268 years.

a) For each variable in the data set, identify the type of variable and describe the summary measures (if any) that you would use to summarise the variable.

b) List the error checks that you would perform on each variable – are there any entries that you would wish to investigate further?

c) What graphical methods would you use to display each of the variables?

d) Basing your answer on the sample of the data that are provided, comment on the likely completeness of the full data set, and on the possible implications of any missing data. What approaches could the authors take to minimise the impact of these missing data?

S2

Individuals with cystic fibrosis (CF) are subject to recurrent respiratory infections (exacerbations) that often require intravenous antibiotic treatment and may result in permanent loss of lung function. Collaco *et al.* (2010) performed a retrospective study on 1535 subjects in the United States to investigate the effects of delivering therapy in hospital and at home. Antibiotic treatment was given following an exacerbation. When raw forced expiratory volume (FEV_1) measurements were converted to Knudson percentiles, the authors found that long-term decline in FEV_1 after exacerbation was observed regardless of whether antibiotics were administered in the hospital (mean = −3.3 and SD = 8.4 percentage points for $n = 602$ courses of therapy) or at home (mean = −3.5 and SD = 7.6 percentage points for $n = 232$ courses of therapy). No significant difference in intervals between courses of antibiotics was observed between hospital (median 119 days, interquartile range 166 (221 – 55) days) and home (median 98 days, interquartile range 155 (204 – 49) days) ($P = 0.29$).

a) Included in the summary of the results is the standard deviation of the decline in FEV_1 for each group. Explain what information the standard deviation conveys and the circumstances in which it would be preferable to quote the standard error of the mean instead of the standard deviation when summarising the results.

b) Determine the standard error of the mean decline in FEV_1 (expressed in percentage points) for both the hospital and home administration of antibiotics.

c) Determine the 95% confidence interval for the mean decline in FEV_1 (expressed in percentage points) for both the hospital and home administration of antibiotics.

d) Interpret the 95% confidence interval for the mean decline in FEV_1 (expressed in percentage points) for the hospital administration of antibiotics.

e) Why do you think the authors provided the median interval between courses of antibiotics rather than the mean interval?

f) Explain what is meant by an interquartile range of 155 days for the home administration of antibiotics.

Collaco JM, Green DM, Cutting GR, Naughton KM, Mogayzel PJ Jr. Location and duration of treatment of cystic fibrosis respiratory exacerbations do not affect outcomes. Am J Respir Crit Care Med 2010; 182: 1137–43.

S3

Malnourishment in elderly patients is associated with an increased risk of adverse clinical events and mortality, and an increased length of hospital stay. Furthermore, persistent malnourishment can lead to deficiencies in various nutritional markers, including vitamins B12 and B6, and folate. O'Leary and colleagues (2011) conducted a cross-sectional study of 52 patients aged ≥60 years who were admitted to a sub-acute geriatric rehabilitation unit in Australia. The aim of the study was to examine associations between the vitamins B12, B6 and folate, homocysteine and methylmalonic acid (MMA), dietary intake, nutritional status and length of stay.

Length of stay was positively correlated with age and MMA (Spearman correlation coefficient (r_s) 0.4, $P < 0.01$ and 0.28, $P < 0.05$, respectively) and negatively correlated with albumin, vitamin B6 and the Mini Nutritional Assessment (MNA) score (r_s −0.35, −0.33 and −0.29, respectively, and $P < 0.05$ for each). When the authors compared subjects whose length of stay was <21 days to subjects whose length of stay was ≥21 days, those with longer lengths of stay were on average, marginally older ($P = 0.054$), had lower vitamin B6 ($P = 0.025$) and lower serum folate concentrations ($P = 0.035$) and had more B vitamin deficiencies ($P = 0.026$) than those with shorter lengths of stay (Table S3.1).

Table S1.1 Portion of data set on cardiovascular disease risk

ID	Entry date	Sex	Age	Ethnic group	Smoking	BMI	TC	HDL-C	TG	LLD	Date of first MI
1	Jun-00	M	36	1	1	25.1	5.6	1.1	3.4	y	
2	Jan-00	M	37	1	0	21.6	.	.	.	n	
3	Mar-00	M	41	1	1	27.2	.	.	.	n	
4	Feb-00	M	34	1	1	21.3	4.0	1.0	0.9	n	
5	Nov-00	M	41	1	2	22.0	5.4	1.8	3.2	n	
6	Sep-00	F	51	1	0	20.5	5.4	1.0	1.1	n	
7	May-00	M	63	1	0	29.4	6.8	1.2	2.6	y	Nov-09
8	Oct-00	F	38	2	0	19.1	3.9	0.9	1.2	n	
9	Aug-00	M	45	3	0	22.1	4.9	0.9	1.7	n	
10	Jul-00	M	38	1	1	21.4	.	.	.	?	
11	Apr-00	M	41	1	2	26.8	.	.	.	.	
12	Feb-00	M	52	1	9	23.4	6.2	1.5	1.2	y	
13	Jun-00	F	50	3	9	23.3	6.8	1.3	2.6	n	
14	Jun-00	M	40	1	0	22.5	3.7	1.4	2.5	n	
15	Mar-00	F	45	1	0	21.9	7.1	1.2	2.9	n	
16	Sep-00	M	50	1	1	24.8	4.9	1.0	1.3	n	
17	Dec-00	F	46	1	2	19.3	5.4	0.9	1.4	y*	
18	Sep-00	F	40	2	2	23.3	5.5	1.9	0.8	.	
19	May-00	F	36	1	0	24.2	5.0	.	.	n	
20	Dec-00	F	51	1	0	23.9	5.1	1.5	1.6	n	
21	Jul-00	M	39	1	0	22.3	6.5	1.0	2.8	n	
22	May-00	M	41	1	9	21.3	4.3	1.2	0.9	n	
23	Jul-00	M	39	9	1	.	5.6	1.6	4.0	.	
24	Jan-00	M	24	2	1	23.0	111.1	.	13.3	y	Aug-03
25	Jul-00	M	35	1	0	19.8	3.1	0.8	0.8	n	
26	Jan-00	M	46	1	0	23.3	5.2	1.2	1.8	n	
27	Feb-00	M	54	2	0	24.6	5.8	3.8	2.1	n	
28	Nov-00	M	44	3	2	.	5.5	1.4	2.3	n	
29	Sep-00	F	43	9	1	24.7	4.8	0.8	2.3	n	
30	Apr-00	F	44	1	0	22.3	3.5	0.7	2.6	n	

Table S3.1 Characteristics of subjects; data shown are mean (standard deviation (SD)) unless otherwise stated. Copyright © 2010, Serdi and Springer Verlag France.

	All subjects	Length of stay	
		<21 days	≥21 days
Number of subjects	54	34	18
Mean length of stay (days)	21 (13)	14 (4)	35 (14)
Age (years)	80 (8)	78 (7)	83 (8)
Body Mass Index (BMI) (kg/m^2)	26.4 (6.8)	26.0 (5.6)	27.4 (8.6)
MNA score	22.2 (3.3)	22.8 (3.0)	21.1 (3.7)
Serum albumin (g/L)	31.8 (4.0)	32.5 (3.7)	30.6 (4.4)
Haemoglobin (g/L)	118 (17)	118 (15)	118 (20)
Lymphocyte count (10^6/L)	1.6 (0.6)	1.6 (0.6)	1.6 (0.7)
Serum folate (nmol/L)	16.8 (7.5)	18.4 (7.4)	13.8 (6.8)
Erythrocyte folate (nmol/L)	1170 (468)	1244 (538)	1051 (303)
Plasma vitamin B6 (nmol/L); median (SD)	17.5 (9.3)	21.5 (9.3)	14.5 (8.3)
Serum vitamin B12 (pmol/L); median (SD)	232 (115)	246 (104)	216 (136)
Plasma MMA (µmol/L); median (SD)	0.22 (0.28)	0.21 (0.16)	0.24 (0.41)
Plasma homocysteine (µmol/L)	15 (5)	14.7 (5.7)	15.5 (3.5)
Number with			
<2 vitamin deficiencies	35	27	8
≥2 vitamin deficiencies	17	7	10

a) Interpret the reported correlations between length of stay and age, MMA and albumin, as well as the results of any significance tests which relate to these correlation coefficients. When would it be most appropriate to display the Spearman correlation coefficient rather than the Pearson correlation coefficient when assessing the association between two values? Is there any evidence to suggest that this was appropriate in this situation?

b) Comment on the way in which the authors have chosen to present the P-values for these correlation coefficients.

c) For most of the variables shown in Table S3.1, the authors chose to present mean values with SDs. For three variables (plasma vitamin B6, serum vitamin B12 and plasma MMA), however, the authors presented medians with standard deviations. Why do you think they presented medians instead of means for these variables? Comment on the appropriateness of presenting standard deviations for these three variables. Finally, comment on the appropriateness of presenting mean values for the other variables in Table S3.1, particularly length of stay. What further information would you like to see to help you answer this question?

d) The authors compared subjects who were hospitalised for <21 days with those hospitalised for ≥21 days. What test(s) would they have used to make comparisons of any numerical variables in Table S3.1? Give reasons for your answers.

e) The authors used a Fisher's exact test to compare the proportion of subjects with <2 or ≥2 vitamin deficiencies between the two groups. Why do you believe that they did this? Using the numbers provided in Table S3.1, investigate whether Fisher's exact test was optimal in this situation. If it was not optimal, what alternative test could have been performed?

O'Leary F, Flood VM, Petocz P, Allman-Farinelli M, Samman S. B vitamin status, dietary intake and length of stay in a sample of elderly rehabilitation patients. J Nutr Health Aging 2011; 15: 485–9.

S4

It has been reported that older individuals experiencing severe burns have a higher mortality rate than younger individuals with severe burns. To assess whether any differences in mortality can be explained by differences in demographic or clinical characteristics of older and younger individuals, Albornoz and colleagues (2011) described a case–control study of 66 patients aged 65 years or older (cases; over-65 group) and 220 patients younger than 65 years (controls; under-65 group) who were admitted with severe burns to the intermediate and intensive care unit of the National Burn Adult Reference Centre in Santiago, Chile. The investigators collected information on the burn agent (e.g. fire or scald), whether inhalation injuries were present, the burn surface area expressed as a percentage of the total body surface area (%TBSA), the deep burn surface area, also expressed as a percentage (%DTBSA), the DTBSA:TBSA proportion and the number of surgeries required to recover the cutaneous barrier. The primary outcomes of the study were the length of stay in the intensive care unit and mortality.

A summary of the characteristics of patients in the two groups is shown in Table S4.1. In unadjusted analyses, the mortality rate was significantly higher in the over-65 group (odds ratio 2.9, 95% confidence interval 1.6–5.2, $P < 0.001$); after controlling for other potential confounders in a multivariable logistic regression analysis, those aged ≥65 years were over 12 times more likely to die from their burns than those in the younger age group (adjusted odds ratio 12.02, $P < 0.001$). The adjusted odds ratio for %TBSA was 1.06 per unit increment ($P < 0.001$), whereas that for the DTBSA:TBSA proportion was 7.6 per unit increment ($P < 0.001$). After adjustment using a multivariable logistic regression analysis, there were no significant associations between mortality and gender, the presence of inhalation injuries or any other comorbidities (e.g. epilepsy, obesity, smoking or cardiovascular disease).

a) Explain why this study cannot be described as a case–control study. What would be a more appropriate description of the study design?

b) Comment on the distributions of the numerical variables summarised in Table S4.1. Do you agree with the authors' choice of summary measures for each variable? If not, what are your reasons for this and what summary measure would you choose to present instead?

c) Using the data provided in Table S4.1, demonstrate how the authors would have calculated the unadjusted odds ratio for mortality.

d) Why did the authors feel that it was important to perform a multivariable logistic regression in this situation? Interpret the adjusted odds ratio provided in the text and its P-value. Why is

Table S4.1 Summary of main characteristics of the over-65 and under-65 groups. Reproduced with permission of Elsevier.

	Age group		P-value
	Over 65	Under 65	
Number of patients	66	220	
Male gender; %	56	75	0.0057
Agent			
Fire; %	70	55	0.01
Scald; %	17	9	0.0005
%TBSA; median (range)	13 (1–76)	22.5 (1–98)	0.0001
%DTBSA; mean (standard deviation)	9.6 (16)	9.2 (16.3)	0.4
Proportion DTBSA:TBSA; mean	41%	23.3%	0.004
Inhalation injury; %	28	43	0.0016
Number of surgeries required; mean	3.7	5.6	0.0003
Mortality; %	48	24	0.0001
Length of stay (days); median (range)	14 (2–126)	15 (1–136)	0.95

the adjusted odds ratio so much higher than the unadjusted odds ratio?

Albornoz CR, Villegas J, Sylvester M, Pena V, Bravo I. Burns are more aggressive in the elderly: proportion of deep burn area/total burn area might have a role in mortality. Burns 2011; 37: 1058–61.

S5

Investigators conducted a randomised controlled trial of two different drugs for the treatment of cryptosporidiosis among children in Uganda. To be eligible for the trial, children were required to have persistent diarrhoea and to have positive stool samples for *Cryptosporidium* spp. Eligible children were randomised on a 1:1 basis to receive either the new drug (Arm A) or standard-of-care (Arm B). A total of 471 children were included in the trial: 243 were randomised to A, and 228 to B. The flowchart (Figure S5.1) shows the flow of children through the trial, as well as the number of children experiencing the primary endpoint (resolution of diarrhoea) by the end of the trial.

a) Comment on the ability of the authors to perform a true intention-to-treat analysis of the primary outcome of this study. What further information would be required to perform such an analysis?

b) The authors chose to perform a modified intention-to-treat analysis; for this analysis, individuals who were lost to follow-up or who died prior to evaluation of the primary endpoint were considered to have not experienced the primary endpoint. Using the figures provided, estimate the treatment effect (odds ratio) for the primary endpoint in the two treatment arms for this population.

c) If the authors now wished to perform a per-protocol (on-treatment) analysis, how would their calculations change? Do the conclusions of their study change in terms of the relative efficacy of the two treatments? What are the limitations of performing such an analysis?

d) Comment on the possible generalisability of their findings to the wider population of children with cryptosporidial diarrhoea who would have met the eligibility criteria for the trial.

S6

Dubbleman *et al.* (2010) compared the effect on the recovery of continence after retropubic radical prostatectomy (RRP) of (i) intensive physiotherapist-guided pelvic floor muscle exercises (PG-PFME) in addition to an information folder with (ii) PFME explained to patients by an information folder only (F-PFME). They postulated that a 10% increase in the proportion of men who regained continence at 6 months with PG-PFME compared with men treated with F-PFME only would constitute a clinically relevant effect. To show statistical significance of this difference at the 5% level with a power of 80% using the Chi-squared test, they determined that 96 men should be randomised to each of the two arms. During the 2-year recruitment period, the number of patients randomised fell short of the target determined by the sample size calculation because of limitations of resources and unexpected changes in treatment preferences. Results were

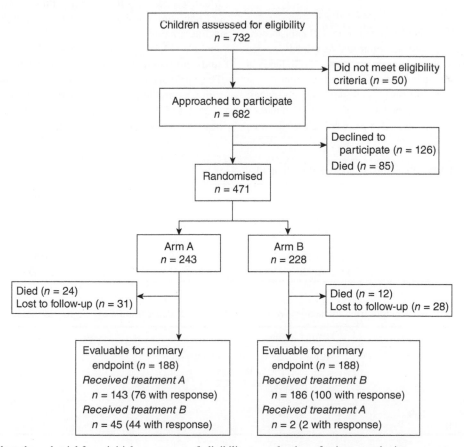

Figure S5.1 Flow of children through trial from initial assessment of eligibility to evaluation of primary endpoint.

available for statistical analysis at 6 months after RRP from only 33 men in each group when 10 (30%) and nine (27%) men had regained continence in the PG-PFME and the F-PFME groups, respectively. The investigators found that this difference was not statistically significant ($P > 0.05$).

a) Explain what is meant by a power of 80%.
b) How does this power relate to the Type II error rate?
c) What was the maximum chance of making a Type I error in this study?
d) If the investigators believed that a 15% increase in the proportion of men who regained continence at 6 months with PG-PFME compared with men treated with F-PFME only would constitute a clinically relevant effect, and if they still decided that they would randomise 96 to each of the two arms, would the power of the study have been greater or less than 80% if the significance level remained at 5%?
e) If the investigators felt that a 1% level of significance would be more appropriate, would the power of the study be greater or less than 80% if the clinically relevant difference was 10% and they intended to randomise 96 men to each arm?
f) Comment on the conclusions. In particular, what other information should the authors have provided to support their conclusions?

Dubbelman Y, Groen J, Wildhagen M, Rikken B, Bosc R. The recovery of urinary continence after radical retropubic prostatectomy: a randomized trial comparing the effect of physiotherapist-guided pelvic floor muscle exercises with guidance by an instruction folder only. BJU Intl. 2010; 106(4): 515–22.

S7

Investigators were interested to know whether vitreal glutamate concentrations were elevated in eyes with anatomic and functional damage from experimental glaucoma. Experimental glaucoma was induced in the right eyes of nine rhesus monkeys by argon laser treatments to the trabecular meshwork. After significant visual field defects and/or typical clinical glaucomatous changes had developed (1.5–13 months), both the left (untreated) and right (treated) eyes were removed, and a sample (0.1–0.2 mL) of posterior vitreous was collected. The investigators performed a statistical test to compare the vitreal glutamate concentrations (µmol/L) in the left (no glaucoma) and right (glaucoma) eyes of the monkeys. The summary values for vitreal glutamate concentrations (based on Carter-Dawson *et al.* 2002) and a computer output of the analysis, similar to that of the SPSS, are shown in Tables S7.1 and S7.2.

a) Which test did the investigators use to compare the vitreal glutamate concentrations in the eyes with and without glaucoma? What alternative test might they have used that would have been appropriate? Explain your reasons for this.
b) What was the null hypothesis for the test that was used?
c) What is the main assumption underlying the test?
d) Explain why you believe the assumption is or is not satisfied.
e) What is meant by a two-tailed test?
f) What is the magnitude of the *P*-value? Interpret it (i.e. explain what it represents).
g) What do you conclude?
h) Interpret the confidence interval found in the computer output.
i) How could you use this confidence interval to test the null hypothesis?

Carter-Dawson L, Crawford ML, Harwerth RS, Smith EL 3rd, Feldman R, Shen FF, Mitchell CK, Whitetree A. Vitreal glutamate concentration in monkeys with experimental glaucoma. Invest Ophthalmol Vis Sci 2002; 43(8): 2633–7.

S8

The PainDETECT questionnaire (PDQ) was developed to classify whether a person's lower back pain is likely to have a neuropathic or non-neuropathic component, based on self-reported pain characteristics (pain pattern, presence of radiating pain and pain quality). Morsø and colleagues (2011) conducted a longitudinal study of participants with low back–related pain in one or both legs. Their primary aim was to investigate whether the PDQ classification was predictive of pain, activity limitation and general health after 3 and 12 months of follow-up. In addition, they wished to describe associations between the PDQ classification at baseline

Table S7.1 Vitreal glutamate concentrations (µmol/L)

	N	Mean	Median	Standard deviation (SD)	Standard error of the mean (SEM)
Left (no glaucoma)	9	5.0889	4.3000	2.09907	.69969
Right (glaucoma)	9	5.7633	4.4000	3.07800	1.02600
Difference (left-right)	9	−.6744	−.1000	3.17008	1.05669
Total	27	3.3926	4.0000	4.00377	.77053

Table S7.2 Computer output from the analysis of the vitreal glutamate concentration data in rhesus monkeys

	Paired differences					t	df	P-value (two-tailed)
	Mean	SD	SEM	95% confidence interval of the difference				
				Lower	Upper			
Difference (no G* − G)	−.674	3.170	1.057	−3.111	1.762	−.638	8	0.541

*G = Glaucoma.

and various measures of pain severity (pain intensity, activity limitation and self-rated general health (measured using a Likert scale from 0 to 10), the need for analgesia and whether the individual had taken any sick leave during the current pain episode) and the individual's psychosocial profile (measured using a Sense of Coherence questionnaire and the Hasenbring Psychosocial Patient Profile).

Of the 145 participants at baseline, 28 (19.3%) were judged to have neuropathic pain according to the PDQ, 77 (53.1%) were judged to have non-neuropathic pain, with the remaining 38 (26.2%) participants having an 'uncertain' classification (two participants could not be classified due to missing data). After excluding those with an uncertain classification, patients with neuropathic pain had worse scores on lower back pain, leg pain, activity limitation, self-rated general health, analgesic use, sick leave and sense of coherence (Table S8.1).

One hundred and thirty-six participants (93.8%) returned questionnaires at 3 months, with 95 (65.5%) returning questionnaires at 12 months. At both time points, responders tended to have higher self-rated general health scores than nonresponders, but no other significant differences were seen between responders and nonresponders. Median self-reported general health scores increased from 2 to 3 from baseline to 3 months in the neuropathic pain group, and from 3 to 4 over the same period in the non-neuropathic pain group, although the overall change itself (both groups combined) was not significant ($P = 0.072$). Median self-reported general health scores did not change further at the 12 month time point.

a) To compare the neuropathic and non-neuropathic pain groups in terms of their sense of coherence at baseline, the authors used a Chi-squared test. What assumption is made when performing this test? Is there any evidence that this assumption is not met?
b) Using the data provided in Table S8.1, perform this Chi-squared test and check that you obtain the same P-value as reported.

c) What other test(s) might be used to compare the baseline sense of coherence between the two groups?
d) One third of individuals failed to return a questionnaire at the 12-month time point. Among those who did complete a follow-up questionnaire at 12 months, there was no change in median self-reported general health score from 3 to 12 months. Why is it important for the authors to ensure that response rates are high? Is there any evidence of attrition bias in this study? If so, what impact is this likely to have on experiencing neuropathic pain?
e) What type of test should the authors use when comparing the change from 3 to 12 months in self-reported general health scores between the two groups? Give your reasons for specifying this type of test.

Morsø L, Kent PM, Albert HB. Are self-reported pain characteristics, classified using the PainDETECT questionnaire, predictive of outcome in people with low back pain and associated leg pain? Clin J Pain 2011; 27(6): 535–41.

S9

Göllner *et al.* (2010) were interested in comparing two loading concepts (immediate loading within the first 24 hours after insertion and conventional loading) on successfully healed and explanted palatal implants in humans in routine practice. The advantages of immediate loading include reduced overall duration of treatment, greater acceptance on the part of patients and better function and aesthetics. The investigators evaluated the histological bone-to-implant contact (BIC) rates in the two loading groups and obtained the following values (all expressed as %):

Immediate functional loading ($n = 10$): 47 98 72 53 93 89 60 79 90 22
Conventional functional loading ($n = 12$): 72 95 65 91 75 86 83 57 78 96 90 100

Table S8.1 Baseline characteristics that were significantly different between the 'neuropathic' and 'non-neuropathic' PDQ groups. Reproduced with permission of Wolters Kluwer Health.

	PainDETECT questionnaire classification		*P*-value
	Neuropathic pain ($n = 28$)	Non-neuropathic pain ($n = 77$)	
Taking analgesia	75.0%	52.0%	0.025
Any sick leave during current episode	59.3%	33.3%	0.044
Sense of coherence*			0.002
Low (1.0–4.4)	42.9%	13.2%	
Below middle (4.5–5.0)	21.4%	22.4%	
Above middle (5.1–5.6)	32.1%	34.2%	
High (5.7–7.0)	3.6%	30.3%	
Hasenbring Psychosocial Patient Profile			0.004
Depressed suppressor	71.4%	31.9%	
Fear avoider	0.0%	7.2%	
Happy suppressor	17.9%	34.8%	
Coper	10.7%	26.1%	
	Median (IQR) (full range)		
Pain intensity (0–10)**			
Back pain	7.0 (5.0–8.8) (0–10)	6.0 (4.0–7.0) (0–9)	0.012
Leg pain	8.0 (5.3–8.0) (0–10)	4.0 (1.0–6.0) (0–9)	0.000
Activity limitation (0–23)**	17.5 (14.3–20.0) (4–23)	10 (7.0–15.0) (1–23)	0.000
Self-rated general health (0–10)*	2.0 (1.0–3.0) (0–5)	3.0 (2.0–4.0) (0–6)	0.001

*High scores are better; **low scores are better.

Table S10.1 The shear bond strength (megapascals) of orthodontic brackets for different drinks

	Group 1: Black tea	Group 2: Mint–lemon herbal tea	Group 3: Mint–maté herbal tea	Group 4: Rosehip fruit tea	Group 5: Coca-Cola (+ve control)	Group 6: Distilled water (−ve control)
	11.39	16.00	9.06	7.24	5.85	9.44
	10.55	16.67	13.83	9.89	5.12	12.56
	13.23	14.60	14.40	7.90	7.79	14.01
	13.39	15.15	10.34	7.11	4.83	12.52
	10.66	10.65	11.83	6.34	5.01	14.52
	11.80	10.57	12.38	6.94	5.45	14.11
	12.44	15.39	14.79	8.43	7.69	12.36
	13.30	15.87	16.30	6.72	5.90	12.67
	12.89	10.37	12.72	6.63	5.24	13.16
	13.28	12.72	12.25	6.76	5.00	12.95
	14.66	9.54	11.46	8.31	5.93	10.81
	11.63	9.08	12.43	8.89	4.42	14.08
	14.50	14.86	15.54	5.51	6.15	14.75
	12.50	11.08	11.20	7.47	6.44	15.22
	10.57	8.61	9.90	8.69	5.65	15.30
Mean	12.45	12.74	12.56	7.52	5.76	13.23
SD	1.33	2.86	2.08	1.15	0.97	1.62

a) Determine the mean and median of the BIC rates in each group. What do their values tell you about the shape of the distribution in each case?

b) Using statistical software or by hand, draw a box plot to show the distributions of the observations in the two groups and explain your findings.

c) What is the most appropriate test to compare the effects of immediate and conventional implant loading on the BIC rates? What is its null hypothesis?

d) Perform this test either using computer software or by hand. What is the P-value, and, hence, what conclusion do you draw about the null hypothesis?

e) What effect might the lack of randomisation have on the conclusions?

f) Provide appropriate summary measures, with confidence intervals, which augment your conclusion about the comparative effectiveness of immediate and conventional loading on the BIC rates.

Göllner P, Jung BA, Kunkel M, Liechti T, Wehrbein H. Immediate vs. conventional loading of palatal implants in humans. Clin Oral Implants Res. 2009; 20(8): 833–7.

S10

Bond failure of brackets during orthodontic treatment is a commonly encountered problem. It has been reported that consumption of acidic soft drinks such as Coca-Cola during orthodontic treatment decreases the retention of brackets. Since herbal teas are now widely consumed world-wide, Ulusoy *et al.* (2009) conducted a study to evaluate the effects of some types of herbal tea on the shear bond strength (SBS) of orthodontic brackets to enamel surfaces. The brackets were bonded with Transbond XT to 90 extracted human premolar teeth and divided randomly into six equally sized groups – four tea (black, mint–maté herbal, mint–lemon herbal, and rosehip fruit) and two control (Coca-Cola and distilled water) groups. On each of 90 consecutive days, all teeth were conditioned with the relevant solution for three 5-minute sessions with equal intervening intervals; for the remainder of the time, they were kept in distilled

water. After 3 months, a shear load was applied directly to each bonded bracket and the load at failure was recorded from which the SBS was determined in megapascals (the lower the SBS value, the poorer the retention). SBS values based on the Ulosoy data, with the estimated mean and standard deviation (SD) for each group, are shown in Table S10.1.

These SBS data were analysed by one-way analysis of variance (ANOVA) followed by *post-hoc* Scheffé multiple comparison tests. If you have the computer facilities, perform these analyses yourself (you can use a different *post-hoc* test if Scheffé's test is not available). Alternatively, consider the results from an SPSS analysis which are shown in Tables S10.2 and S10.3.

a) What is the null hypothesis for the one-way ANOVA?

b) What are the assumptions underlying this test? If you have computer facilities, check out these assumptions. Are they satisfied? If they are not satisfied, which test would you have performed instead to compare the groups? What is its null hypothesis?

c) What do you conclude from the ANOVA table?

d) Why is it customary to perform a *post hoc* comparison test, such as the Scheffé test, to compare each pair of groups?

e) What do you conclude from the Scheffé test results? How do you think your conclusions might have altered if pairwise comparisons had been undertaken using a series of unpaired *t*-tests instead of the Scheffé (or similar) *post hoc* tests?

Table S10.2 One-way ANOVA table for the shear bond strength data

ANOVA					
SBS					
	Sum of squares	df	Mean square	F	P-value
Between groups	773.821	5	154.764	48.421	<0.001
Within groups	268.481	84	3.196		
Total	1042.302	89			

Table S10.3 Scheffé's test results for the shear bond strength data (I and J are labels to identify the groups that are being compared)

	(I) group	(J) group	Mean difference (I–J)	P-value	95% confidence interval	
					Lower bound	Upper bound
Scheffé	1	2	−.29074	0.999	−2.5156	1.9341
		3	−.11041	>0.999	−2.3353	2.1145
		4	4.93079	<0.001	2.7059	7.1557
		5	6.68839	<0.001	4.4635	8.9133
		6	−.77891	0.920	−3.0038	1.4460
	2	3	.18033	>0.999	−2.0446	2.4052
		4	5.22153	<0.001	3.9966	7.4464
		5	6.97913	<0.001	4.7542	9.2040
		6	−.48817	0.989	−2.7131	1.7367
	3	4	5.04120	<0.001	2.8163	7.2661
		5	6.79879	<0.001	4.5739	9.0237
		6	−.66850	0.958	−2.8934	1.5564
	4	5	1.75759	0.215	−.4673	3.9825
		6	−5.70970	<0.001	−7.9346	−3.4848
	5	6	−7.46729	<0.001	−9.6922	−5.2424

f) Although this experiment could not completely replicate the complex oral environment, the authors of the original paper believed that it confirmed that Coca-Cola and rosehip fruit tea may each be a causative factor in bracket – enamel bonding failure. Do you agree?

Ulusoy C, Müjdeci A and Gökay O. The effect of herbal teas on the shear bond strength of orthodontic brackets. Eur J Orthod 2009; 31: 385–9.

S11

The mortality associated with ruptured abdominal aortic aneurysm (rAAA) has decreased by 3.5% per decade over the last 50 years to a rate in 2010 of 40–50%. Reports have indicated that endovascular repair (EVAR) is feasible for rAAA and may offer potential benefits over open repair. With a view to assessing this, Davenport *et al.* (2010) performed a retrospective observational study using the 2005–7 American College of Surgeons National Surgical Quality Improvement Program (ACS NSQIP) database in which surgeon preference determined the type of repair performed. The authors compared the 30-day outcomes for EVAR versus open rAAA repair in 427 patients of whom 328 (76.8%) underwent open repair. The number of patients dying within the first 30 days was 22 in those patients with EVAR and 123 in those with open rAAA.

a) Construct a contingency table of the results.
b) What percentage of patients died within 30 days in each group?
c) Assuming that the investigators have information on 30-day outcomes of all patients on the database, which test should be used to compare the 30-day mortality in the two groups and what is its null hypothesis?
d) What is (are) the assumption(s) underlying this test? Is (are) it (they) satisfied?
e) If you have access to a statistical package on a computer, use it to compare the mortality in the two groups. Alternatively, perform the test by hand using the appropriate formula for the test statistic and refer its value to the relevant probability distribution to

Table S12.1 Improvement in preparedness over time: percentage response to the statement. © 2007 Cave, *et al.*, licensee BioMed Central Ltd.

Year of survey	Agree or strongly agree	Neither agree nor disagree	Disagree or strongly disagree
	n (%)	n (%)	n (%)
2000–2001	1111 (36.2)	689 (22.5)	1262 (41.3)
2003	1382 (50.3)	519 (18.9)	844 (30.8)
2005	1195 (58.5)	533 (26.1)	308 (15.3)

obtain a P-value. What is the value of the test statistic, what distribution does it follow and what is the P-value?
f) What conclusions do you draw about the 30-day mortality with EVAR compared to that with open rAAA? Explain any reservations you might have concerning this conclusion.
g) What additional numerical information should be provided to give a full and useful description of the results?

Davenport DL, O'Keeffe SD, Minion DJ, Sorial EE, Endean ED, Xenos ES. Thirty-day NSQIP database outcomes of open versus endoluminal repair of ruptured abdominal aortic aneurysms. J Vasc Surg 2010; 51(2): 305–9.

S12

In response to findings that newly qualified doctors in the United Kingdom felt unprepared by their medical school for their first medical posts, the UK General Medical Council recommended that medical schools should improve their preparation of students for the first year of working life. As a result, all medical schools in the United Kingdom made curricular changes to bring their courses in line with recommendations, although the timing of these changes varied substantially. In order to investigate the impact of these changes on the way newly qualified doctors feel, Cave and colleagues (2007) conducted a questionnaire survey of newly qualified doctors in the United Kingdom in 2000, 2001, 2003 and 2005. The questionnaires were sent to doctors approximately 9 months after their graduations. For the purposes of the analyses, the authors combined the 2000 and 2001 cohorts, as the 2001 cohort had included only a random sample of 25% of those qualifying in that year. Respondents were asked to state their level of agreement with the statement 'My experience at medical school has prepared me well for the jobs I have undertaken so far' on a five-point scale from 'strongly agree' to 'strongly disagree'.

Questionnaires were sent to 5330 doctors in 2000–2001, 4257 doctors in 2003 and 2784 doctors in 2005; response rates were 67%, 65% and 43% respectively. The authors noted that in the 2005 survey, graduates of one particular medical school were under-represented, but there were no other significant differences in response rate by region or method of distribution. Female doctors were, however, significantly more likely to respond ($P < 0.001$) than male doctors. The results are shown in Table S12.1. The Chi-squared test for a linear trend in the proportion that agreed or strongly agreed with the statement gave a P-value of <0.001 (Chi-squared value = 259.5, $df = 1$).

Overall, 12 medical schools implemented new courses between 1999 and 2004, with eight making changes from 1999 to 2002, and four making changes after 2002 (Table S12.2). Schools that made their changes from 1999 to 2002 experienced a large increase in the

Table S12.2 Changes in preparedness when new courses were introduced: proportion (%) strongly agreeing or agreeing that their medical school prepared them well. © 2007 Cave, *et al.*, licensee BioMed Central Ltd.

Period of course change	Year of survey		
	2000–2001	2003	2005
1999–2002 (8 schools)	250/859 (29.1%)	563/985 (57.2%)	549/826 (66.4%)
2002–2004 (4 schools)	119/468 (25.4%)	207/508 (40.7%)	187/337 (55.4%)

proportion that strongly agreed or agreed with the statement from the 2000/2001 cohort to the 2003 cohort, with a smaller increase to the 2005 cohort. The pattern seen among schools that made their changes from 2002 onwards was less clear-cut.

a) Explain why the authors chose to perform a Chi-squared test for trend when investigating the association between the year of the survey and the proportion of doctors who agreed or strongly agreed with the statement. Using the information provided in the text and Table S12.1, show that the value of the Chi-squared test statistic for trend is 259.5, as the authors report.

b) Female doctors were more likely to respond than male doctors. Is it possible that this might introduce bias into the assessment of time trends? How could the authors investigate this?

c) The authors informally described the differences in trends in the percentage of doctors strongly agreeing or agreeing with the statement between schools that changed their course from 1999 to 2002 and those that changed their course from 2002 to 2004. If the authors had wished to test formally whether these trends differed, what test(s) might they have performed?

d) What are your concerns, if any, about combining the data from the different schools in this way? What additional comparisons might you consider to alleviate your concerns?

Cave J, Goldacre M, Lambert T, Woolf K, Jones A, Dacre J. Newly qualified doctors' views about whether their medical school had trained them well: questionnaire surveys. BMC Medical Education 2007; 7: 38.

S13

Accurate measurement of children's weight is rarely possible in paediatric resuscitation, and rapid estimates are made to ensure appropriate drug and fluid doses and equipment selection. Weight is commonly estimated from formulae based on children's age, or from their height using the Broselow tape. Cattermole *et al.* (2010) investigated the relationship of age, height, foot-length and mid-arm circumference (MAC) with weight in healthy Hong Kong children in order to derive an optimal weight-estimation formula. Amongst 448 children aged 9–11, they found that MAC (measured in cm) had the strongest relationship with weight (measured in kg). The estimated Pearson correlation coefficient was 0.91 (95% CI 0.90–0.93) and the estimated linear regression line was given by: Weight = −29.14 + 2.94MAC.

a) What is the intercept of the regression line? Interpret its value and comment.

b) What is the slope of the estimated regression line? Interpret its value.

Table S14.1 Estimated partial regression coefficients from a multiple regression analysis investigating the relationship between upper airway length and the Respiratory Disturbance Index. Reproduced with permission of Elsevier.

	Coefficient	*P*-value
Age (years)	0.2	0.52
Gender (male – reference)	−21.1	0.04
BMI (kg/m^2)	0.7	0.43
UAL (mm)	3.5	<0.001
HMP (mm)	−0.7	0.30
Soft palate length (PNS-SP, mm)	−0.8	0.24

c) The 95% confidence interval for the Pearson correlation coefficient was 0.90 to 0.93. What does this mean?

d) Is the slope of the regression line significantly different from zero (explain your answer)?

e) Assuming that the assumptions underlying the regression model are satisfied, do you believe that the regression line is a good fit to the data (explain your reasoning)?

Cattermole GN, Leung PYM, Mak PSK. Mid-arm circumference can be used to estimate children's weights. Resuscitation 2010; 81: 1105–10.

S14

Susarla *et al.* (2010) measured the upper airway length (UAL) on lateral cephalograms in order to assess its effect on the Respiratory Disturbance Index (RDI), indicating the severity of obstructive sleep apnoea (OSA). The RDI is based on the total number of complete cessations (apnoea) and partial obstructions (hypopnoea) of breathing occurring per hour of sleep. These pauses in breathing must last for 10 seconds and are associated with a decrease in oxygenation of the blood. In general, the RDI can be used to classify the severity of disease (mild 5–15, moderate >15–30 and severe >30 events per hour). The investigators enrolled 96 adult subjects (76 males) with OSA, and in these subjects the RDI ranged from an average of 1.9 to 160 per hour. The UAL was measured as the distance (mm) parallel to the long axis of the airway, between a horizontal plane tangent to the superior aspect of the hyoid bone and a horizontal plane tangent to the posterior palate. Pearson correlation coefficients were computed to identify associations between disease severity (RDI) and each of the demographic (age, height, weight and BMI) and cephalometric variables (UAL, PAS, HMP and PNS-SP). Associations with $P \leq 0.15$ in bivariate analyses and biologically relevant measures (i.e., age, gender and BMI) were included in a multiple linear regression model to evaluate the adjusted association between UAL and RDI. For the multiple regression analysis, $P \leq 0.05$ was considered statistically significant. The estimated partial regression coefficients of this multiple regression model (for which $R^2 = 0.6$) and their associated *P*-values are shown in Table S14.1.

a) The authors included six covariates in the model. Explain why you think this was or was not an acceptable number of covariates.

b) What do you conclude from the results shown in Table S14.1?

c) Explain the meaning of the estimated partial regression coefficient for UAL.

d) Explain the meaning of the estimated partial regression coefficient for gender.

e) What additional information would you like to see if you want to understand the implications of the model fully?

f) The authors provide some information about how much of the variability in RDI is accounted for by this model. What is the value of their estimate? What would be a better indicator of this variability?

g) What are the assumptions underlying the regression model, and how can they be checked? What would be the implications if they are not satisfied?

Susarla SM, Abramson ZR, Dodson TB, Kaban LB. Cephalometric measurement of upper airway length correlates with the presence and severity of obstructive sleep apnea. J Oral Maxillofac Surg 2010; 68(11): 2846–55.

S15

Clark *et al.* (2011) performed a retrospective cohort study to evaluate the baseline renal function of patients with chronic kidney disease (CKD) who underwent partial nephrectomy for renal tumours. Stage III CKD was present if the patient had an estimated glomerular filtration rate (eGFR) from 30 to 59 ml/minute/1.73 m^2, with values lower than 30 indicating a higher stage of kidney disease. Two hundred and eighty of the 952 patients with Stages I or II CKD at baseline (eGFR $\geq$60 ml/minute/1.73 m^2) developed at least Stage III CKD at follow-up of between 3 and 18 months after partial nephrectomy. The authors used linear logistic regression analysis to investigate the association of newly acquired CKD Stage III or greater with pertinent demographic, tumour and surgical factors. The presence of comorbid conditions such as coronary artery disease, diabetes mellitus or hypertension was not statistically significant. The statistically significant factors are shown in Table S15.1.

a) Interpret the odds ratio for age.

b) Interpret the odds ratio for gender.

c) Interpret the odds ratio for preoperative eGFR.

d) Provide a statement which incorporates all these findings to explain the effect of these factors on eGFR.

e) If you were not given the *P*-value for the odds ratio for any one of these factors, how would you be able to assess whether or not that factor had a significant effect on progression to at least Stage III CKD?

f) Why could the use of logistic regression analysis in these circumstances be criticised? What alternative way of analysing the data might the investigators have used in order to assess the independent effect of these factors on progression to at least Stage III CKD?

Clark MA, Shikanov S, Raman JD, Smith B, Kaag M, Russo P, Wheat JC, Wolf JS Jr, Matin SF, Huang WC, Shalhav AL, Eggener SE. Chronic kidney disease before and after partial nephrectomy. Urology 2011; 185(1): 43–8.

S16

Osteoporotic fractures are common in elderly women and are associated with high healthcare costs and increased suffering. Although the risk of osteoporotic fractures is greater in those with low calcium levels, the optimal level of calcium intake to prevent osteoporosis and fractures is unclear. To study the association between dietary intake of calcium and the risk of fractures (of any type, and of hip fractures specifically), Warensjo and colleagues (2011) used data from the Swedish Mammography Cohort, a large, population-based prospective study of Swedish women. The cohort was established in 1987–1990 and includes women residing in two Swedish counties (Uppsala and Västmanland) who had been born in the years 1914–1948. Women completed a food frequency questionnaire at baseline (1987–1990) and a second expanded questionnaire in 1997. The present study included information on 61 433 women with baseline data, of whom 38 084 also provided data in 1997. Information on fracture events was captured via linkage with the Swedish National Patient Registry and from outpatient registers. For each participant, follow-up time was accrued from baseline until the date of fracture, date of death, date of leaving the study regions or end of the study period (31 December 2008). Average calcium intake was calculated based on the information provided from the two dietary questionnaires and was stratified into quintiles. Estimates of age-adjusted and multivariable-adjusted hazard ratios (HRs) were obtained using Cox proportional hazards regression analysis.

Over a median of 19.2 years of follow-up (with a total of 996 800 person-years at risk), 14 738 women (24%) experienced a new fracture (any type) of whom 3871 (6%) experienced a new hip fracture. Fracture rates stratified by the calcium quintile are shown in Table S16.1, as are the mean (standard deviation (SD)) age of women in each quintile group.

a) Describe the association between average cumulative calcium intake and first (any and hip) fracture risk. Given the variation in age in the different quintile groups, what impact do you think this will have on the relative hazard estimates for each quintile (when expressed relative to the third quintile)?

b) Using the third quintile (882–996 mg) as the reference group, calculate the unadjusted relative rates for the remaining four quintile groups for first (any) fracture. Do these differ substantially from the age-adjusted HRs reported in Table S16.1 (noting that although the authors report HRs from a Cox proportional hazards regression model, these should be similar to relative rates in this situation)? Is this what you would expect based on your answer to (a)?

c) Do the results suggest that there may be a linear association between average cumulative calcium intake and first (any) fracture risk?

d) Repeat the analyses in (b) and (c) for first (hip) fractures – how do your results differ from those for first (any) fractures?

Table S15.1 Estimated odds ratios derived from a linear logistic regression analysis to investigate the relationship between CKD Stage III and potential risk factors

	Estimated odds ratio (95% CI)	*P*-value
Age (per year)	1.05 (1.03 to 1.07)	<0.001
Gender (male – reference)	1.79 (1.25 to 2.56)	0.002
Tumour size (per cm)	1.20 (1.06 to 1.35)	0.003
Clamping of renal artery alone or renal artery and vein (artery alone – reference)	2.16 (1.06 to 4.41)	0.035
Preoperative eGFR (per ml/ min/1.73 m^2)	0.95 (0.94 to 0.97)	<0.001

Table S16.1 Rate of first fracture (any or hip) by quintiles of average cumulative intake of dietary calcium in the cohort, as well as mean (standard deviation (SD)) age at entry in the cohort. Reproduced with permission of BMJ Publishing Group Ltd.

	Quintile				
	1	2	3	4	5
Calcium intake (mg)	<751	751–882	882–996	996–1137	>1137
Age (years) at entry; mean (SD)	54.4 (10.0)	53.8 (9.8)	53.5 (9.7)	53.3 (9.6)	53.6 (9.6)
First fracture (any)					
Number of fractures	3243	2941	2841	2872	2841
Person-years at risk	188 850	199 411	202 680	203 216	202 656
Rate per 1000 person-years	17.2	14.7	14.0	14.1	14.0
(95% confidence interval (CI))	(16.6, 17.8)	(14.2, 15.3)	(13.5, 14.5)	(13.6, 14.7)	(13.5, 14.5)
Age-adjusted hazard ratio (HR)	1.25	1.06	1.0 (reference)	1.00	1.00
(95% CI)	(1.19, 1.32)	(1.00, 1.11)		(0.96, 1.06)	(0.95, 1.06)
Adjusted HR	1.18	1.04	1.0 (reference)	1.02	1.00
(95% CI)[1]	(1.12, 1.25)	(0.98, 1.10)		(0.96, 1.07)	(0.95, 1.06)
First fracture (hip)					
Number of fractures	956	751	680	730	754
Person-years at risk	205 895	214 001	217 223	217 228	215 638
Rate per 1000 person-years	4.6	3.5	3.1	3.4	3.5
(95% CI)	(4.4, 4.9)	(3.3, 3.8)	(2.9, 3.4)	(3.1, 3.6)	(3.3, 3.8)
Age-adjusted HR	1.51	1.13	1.0 (reference)	1.07	1.12
(95% CI)	(1.37, 1.67)	(1.01, 1.24)		(0.97, 1.19)	(1.01, 1.24)
Adjusted HR	1.29	1.09	1.0 (reference)	1.13	1.19
(95% CI)[1]	(1.17, 1.43)	(0.98, 1.21)		(1.01, 1.26)	(1.06, 1.32)

[1]Adjusted for age, total energy, retinol, alcohol intake, vitamin D intake, Body Mass Index, height, nulliparity, educational level, physical activity level, smoking status, calcium supplementation, previous fracture of any type before baseline and Charlson's comorbidity index.

e) The authors also re-fitted the model incorporating the cumulative calcium intake as a continuous covariate (rather than categorising it into quintiles). The fully adjusted HR of any first fracture associated with a 300 mg higher calcium level was estimated as 0.94 (95% confidence interval 0.92, 0.96). Explain how the HR is interpreted. The authors now wish to re-scale the HR so that the estimate relates to a 200 mg higher calcium level. Explain how they would go about doing this, and use the value of 0.94 to obtain an approximate estimate of this re-scaled value together with its 95% confidence interval.

Warensjo E, Buberg L, Melhus H, Gedeborg R, Mallmin H, Wolk A, Michaelsson K. Dietary calcium intake and risk of fracture and osteoporosis: prospective longitudinal cohort study. BMJ 2011; 342: d1473.

S17

To identify the rate of and risk factors for falls among licenced thoroughbred racing jockeys in Australia, Hitchens and colleagues (2011) collated data from three states (Victoria, South Australia and Tasmania). A fall was defined as a rider being dislodged from a horse, regardless of the outcome, and an injury was considered to have occurred if the jockey was declared unfit to ride or was taken to hospital after the fall. Data were available for every race conducted at race meetings run by a Principal Racing Authority from 1 August 2002 to 31 July 2009. The authors used Poisson regression to estimate incidence rate ratios (IRRs) with 95% confidence intervals; the logarithm of the number of rides was included as an offset in the model. Analyses were stratified by the type of race (hurdle or steeplechase).

Table S17.1 shows information for the steeplechase races only.

a) Using the data provided in Table S17.1, calculate the fall rates (expressed per 100 rides) for the different jump types and for the different race distances.

b) With this information, calculate the unadjusted IRRs compared to 'standard' for jump type and to '<3500 m' for race distances, ensuring that you obtain the same values as in Table S17.1.

c) If the authors had only presented unadjusted IRRs, what conclusions would they have reached regarding the associations between the fall rate and the different jump types and race distances? Explain your reasoning.

d) Is there any evidence that the presence of confounding might change the authors' conclusions from part (c)? Explain your answer.

e) The authors combined data for the number of jump races that the horse had previously started ('previous starts') and for the number of horses in the race ('field size'). Why do you think they did this? Is there any statistical evidence that the effect of field size on the fall rate varies according to the number of previous starts by the horse? What additional test would you perform to answer this question formally?

Hitchens P, Blizzard L, Jones G, Day L, Fell J. Predictors of race-day jockey falls in jumps racing in Australia. Accid Anal Prevent 2011; 43: 840–7.

S18

Oster and colleagues (2011) used data from the Pediatric Health Information System (PHIS) database to describe the associations between racial or ethnic disparities and access to care and mortality among children undergoing surgery for congenital heart disease. In particular, they were interested in whether any racial or ethnic differences in mortality rates could be *explained* by differences in access to care between those of different ethnic or racial origin. The PHIS is a large, multicentre administrative database; participating paediatric tertiary care hospitals contribute information

Table S17.1 Number of falls and rides, incidence rate ratios (IRRs) for steeplechase racing. Reproduced with permission of Elsevier.

Study factor	Falls	Rides	Unadjusted IRR (95% CI)	Adjusted* IRR (95% CI)
Jump type				
Standard	133	1253	1.00	1.00
Mark II	12	141	0.80 (0.46, 1.41)	0.74 (0.44, 1.13)
Mark III	80	1366	0.55 (0.42, 0.72)	0.51 (0.42, 0.63)
Club level				
Country	32	326	1.00	1.00
Provincial	112	1382	0.83 (0.57, 1.20)	0.81 (0.57, 1.14)
Metropolitan	81	1052	0.78 (0.53, 1.16)	0.68 (0.46, 1.01)
Jockey licence				
Licence A	168	2222	1.00	1.00
Licence B	57	535	1.41 (1.03, 1.92)	1.49 (1.21, 1.84)
Race distance (m)				
<3500	150	1881	1.00	1.00
3500–3999	40	594	0.84 (0.60, 1.18)	0.76 (0.56, 1.02)
≥4000	35	285	1.54 (1.08, 2.19)	1.17 (0.87, 1.58)
Previous rides this meeting				
0	134	1883	1.00	1.00
1	73	717	1.43 (1.08, 1.89)	1.21 (0.99, 1.48)
≥2	18	160	1.58 (0.97, 2.57)	1.26 (0.88, 1.80)
Prize money				
≤$10 000	65	708	1.00	1.00
$10 001–20 000	41	620	0.72 (0.51, 1.03)	0.74 (0.56, 0.98)
$20 001–50 000	33	574	0.63 (0.43, 0.92)	0.69 (0.50, 0.95)
>$50 000	86	858	1.09 (0.82, 1.46)	1.17 (0.83, 1.64)
Previous starts by horse and field size				
<5 starts				
<8 starters	7	144	1.00	1.00
8–12 starters	34	287	2.44 (1.19, 4.99)	2.46 (1.41, 4.30)
>12 starters	7	45	3.20 (1.27, 8.04)	4.51 (2.17, 9.34)
5–9 starts				
<8 starters	12	204	1.21 (0.53, 2.75)	1.35 (0.72, 2.55)
8–12 starters	37	538	1.41 (0.70, 2.88)	1.78 (1.01, 3.12)
>12 starters	15	123	2.51 (1.14, 5.52)	3.19 (1.69, 6.02)
≥10 starts				
<8 starters	28	322	1.79 (0.86, 3.71)	2.04 (1.16, 3.59)
8–12 starters	63	917	1.41 (0.71, 2.81)	1.85 (1.07, 3.19)
>12 starters	22	180	2.51 (1.19, 5.31)	3.00 (1.62, 5.53)

*Adjusted for all other variables in the table.

to the database on demographics, diagnoses, procedures, interventions and outcomes for all inpatient encounters among children. The primary outcome for the study was in-hospital death after congenital heart surgery. The main predictor of interest was a combined measure of race and ethnicity (classified as Hispanic, non-Hispanic white, non-Hispanic black or other non-Hispanic, with patients with missing race excluded). The authors fitted two multivariable models: the first included adjustment for the child's age (<30 days, 30 days–1 year or >1 year), sex, whether a genetic syndrome was present and the surgery risk category (an ordinal categorical variable with values from 1 to 6 that provides a measure of the 'risk' associated with each surgical encounter); the second included additional adjustment for access to care, as captured through variables for insurance type (government, private or other) and hospital of surgery. Analyses were performed using Poisson regression, with robust variance estimation to allow for the fact that some children underwent more than one episode of surgery.

The 44 017 eligible children in the database provided information on a total of 49 833 congenital heart surgery encounters at 41 children's hospitals. Overall in-hospital mortality over the study period (2004 to 2008) was 3.4%. Unadjusted mortality rates were 2.8% among the 26 287 non-Hispanic whites, 3.6% among the 6142 non-Hispanic blacks, 3.9% among the 8686 Hispanics and 4.6% among the 6691 other non-Hispanics. The key findings from the Poisson regression analysis are shown in Table S18.1.

a) Interpret the results of the baseline-adjusted model. Is there any evidence of racial differences in mortality rates based on these data?
b) The authors have selected the non-Hispanic white group as the reference category for this analysis. Had they instead selected the Hispanic group as the reference group, what would be the effect on the reported RR values for the non-Hispanic white, non-Hispanic black and other non-Hispanic ethnic groups?
c) To address their question of whether any differences in mortality rates between those of different ethnic or racial groups could

Table S18.1 Adjusted in-hospital mortality risk ratios (RR) and confidence intervals (CI) after congenital heart surgery, 2004–2008. Reproduced with permission of Elsevier.

Race or ethnicity	Baseline adjustment[1]			Full adjustment[2]		
	RR	95% CI	*P*-value	RR	95% CI	*P*-value
Non-Hispanic white	1.00	–	–	1.00	–	–
Non-Hispanic black	1.32	1.14, 1.52	0.0002	1.27	1.09, 1.47	0.0021
Other non-Hispanic	1.41	1.25, 1.60	<0.0001	1.56	1.37, 1.78	<0.0001
Hispanic	1.21	1.07, 1.37	0.0028	1.22	1.05, 1.41	0.0073

[1]Adjusted for age, sex, genetic syndrome and surgery risk category.
[2]Adjusted for age, sex, genetic syndrome, surgery risk category and access to care (insurance type and hospital of surgery).

be explained by differences in access to care between the groups, the authors additionally adjusted for two measures that captured access to care. Under the hypothesis that access to care completely explained any racial differences, what values for the RRs would the authors have expected to see in the fully adjusted model? Are their results consistent with this hypothesis?

d) Describe any limitations in the approach that the authors have taken in using the fully adjusted model.

e) The authors used robust variance estimation to allow for the fact that some children underwent more than one episode of surgery. Why did they do this? If they had not done this, what would have been the effect on the confidence intervals and *P*-values reported in Table S18.1?

Oster ME, Strickland MJ, Mahle WT. Racial and ethnic disparities in postoperative mortality following congenital heart surgery. J Pediatr 2011; 159(2): 222–6.

S19

The association between birth weight (BW) and systolic blood pressure (SBP) levels in later life has been considered in the past to provide some of the strongest, and most consistent, support for the 'foetal origins' hypothesis of adult disease. A 1996 paper based on 28 retrospective studies estimated (without making any allowance for the size of the studies) that a 1 kg higher BW is typically associated with a 2–4 mm Hg lower SBP. Huxley *et al.* (2002) investigated these 28 and a further 27 studies that reported regression coefficients for this association: 52 of the 55 studies reported lower SBP associated with higher BW. Ordering these studies according to their size yielded a clear trend towards weaker associations in the larger studies. There were an additional 58 studies (23 of which did not observe a relationship between SBP and BW) that did not report regression coefficients and were not included in the overall assessment of the association. BW was obtained mostly from birth records, but parental recall or self-reports of BW also provided information on BW in some cases. Huxley *et al.* investigated the possibility of various biases occurring and were concerned about the impact of random error, publication bias, measurement error, confounders and an inappropriate adjustment for current weight. Their findings suggested that BW is of little relevance to SBP in later life. In the context of this study:

a) Explain what is meant by random error.
b) Explain what is meant by publication bias.

c) Explain what is meant by measurement error.
d) Explain what is meant by confounding. Do you think confounding might have been a problem in the original investigation? Explain your answer.
e) Can you explain why it might be inappropriate to adjust for current weight?

Huxley R, Neil A, Collins R. Unravelling the fetal origins hypothesis: is there really an inverse association between birth weight and subsequent blood pressure? Lancet 2002; 360: 659–65.

S20

There have been several review articles that have shown a relationship between shorter sleep duration and an increased risk of obesity in children. However, many of the studies included in these reviews were cross-sectional or were methodologically flawed, either because they failed to use objective measures of sleep duration or because they failed to take account of changes in sleep patterns over time. To determine the relation between serial measures of sleep and subsequent body composition in young children, Carter and colleagues (2011) conducted a longitudinal study of 244 children who were participating in a birth cohort (the Family Lifestyle, Activity, Movement and Eating (FLAME) study) in New Zealand. The children were followed from the age of 3 years, with annual measures of diet, sleep and physical activity recorded at ages 3, 4 and 5 years.

The authors wished to describe the association between duration of sleep (hours/day) and Body Mass Index (BMI) at each annual visit. To make maximum use of the data collected, they used a mixed-effects (also called a 'random-effects') regression model with random effects for the child and his or her age; this allowed them to incorporate the repeated measurements from each child and also permitted BMI to increase with age at a different rate from child to child. The authors fitted a series of univariable models, which considered the associations between BMI and sleep duration plus other variables thought to be associated with BMI in children (age, sex, maternal education and income, maternal BMI, ethnicity, child's birth weight and whether the mother smoked during pregnancy). The authors also fitted models that assessed associations between BMI and behavioural factors including physical activity, television viewing, fruit and vegetable intake and noncore foods intake. After fitting univariable models, the authors fitted a series of multivariable models. The first (model 1) adjusted the association between BMI and sleep duration for the child's age and sex only, the second (model 2) additionally adjusted

Table S20.1 Results of random effects models that assess the association between Body Mass Index (BMI) and duration of sleep at ages 3, 4 and 5 years. Reproduced with permission of BMJ Publishing Group Ltd.

Factor	Univariate model	Multivariable models		
		Model 1	Model 2	Model 3
Age (years)	−0.11 (−0.16, −0.08)	−0.32 (−0.38, −0.27)	−0.33 (−0.38, −0.27)	−0.33 (−0.39, −0.28)
Sex (male)	0.24 (−0.08, 0.57)	0.13 (−0.21, 0.46)	0.07 (−0.25, 0.38)	0.04 (−0.28, 0.37)
Maternal education (high)	−0.18 (−0.51, 0.16)	–	−0.00 (−0.34, 0.33)	−0.03 (−0.38, 0.32)
Maternal BMI	0.03 (0.00, 0.06)	–	0.03 (−0.00, 0.06)	0.03 (−0.00, 0.05)
Income (6 categories)	−0.10 (−0.21, 0.00)	–	−0.04 (−0.15, 0.07)	0.03 (−0.14, 0.08)
Ethnicity (Maori)*	1.22 (0.72, 1.73)	–	0.97 (0.46, 1.47)	0.95 (0.44, 1.45)
Ethnicity (Pacific)*	0.16 (−0.68, 0.99)	–	−0.47 (−1.34, 0.39)	−0.43 (−1.32, 0.47)
Birth weight (kg)	0.12 (−0.23, 0.47)	–	0.32 (−0.03, 0.67)	0.32 (−0.04, 0.68)
Smoking during pregnancy (yes)	0.89 (0.50, 1.28)	–	0.82 (0.41, 1.23)	0.79 (0.38, 1.21)
Physical activity (1 SD counts/min)	0.06 (−0.16, 0.28)	–	–	−0.02 (−0.24, 0.20)
TV viewing (hours/day)	0.21 (−0.00, 0.43)	–	–	0.11 (−0.11, 0.32)
Fruit and vegetable intake (servings/day)	0.05 (−0.08, 0.17)	–	–	0.09 (−0.03, 0.22)
Noncore foods intake (servings/day)	0.14 (0.00, 0.29)	–	–	0.03 (−0.11, 0.18)
Sleep (hours/day)	**−0.38 (−0.70, −0.07)**	**−0.37 (−0.69, −0.05)**	**−0.24 (−0.55, 0.10)**	**−0.25 (−0.56, 0.06)**

Figures are estimates for change in BMI associated with a one-unit change in independent variables (univariate model) and adjusted for the other variables (multivariable models).

for maternal and pregnancy factors and the third (model 3) additionally adjusted for the behavioural factors (Table S20.1).

a) Why did the authors choose to perform a mixed-effects regression model in this situation? Why would a simple linear regression model not have been optimal? What are the different 'levels' in the data set?

b) Describe the reported association between the duration of sleep and BMI obtained from the univariable model. Is this association likely to be statistically significant? Explain your answer.

c) Is there any evidence that the association between sleep and BMI is confounded by other factors? If so, explain why this is the case and what factors may be responsible.

d) Overall, do you conclude that there is a strong association between the duration of sleep and a child's BMI in this study? Explain the reason for your answer.

e) What other factors appear to have an influence on a child's BMI in this study?

Carter PK, Taylor BJ, Williams SM, Taylor RW. Longitudinal analysis of sleep in relation to BMI and body fat in children: the FLAME study. BMJ 2011; 342: d2712.

S21

It has been reported that the combination of on-demand sedation and a novel water method for aiding colonoscope insertion permitted 52% of a cohort of 44 veterans to complete colonoscopy without requiring sedation. Leung *et al.* (2010) conducted a randomised controlled trial to investigate this finding. They wanted to assess if, compared with the air method, the water method increased the proportion of patients being able to complete colonoscopy without sedation. They were also interested in comparing other variables in the two groups, such as the maximum discomfort experienced during colonoscopy (measured on a scale of 0 = 'no discomfort' to 10 = 'severe discomfort').

One hundred veterans were randomised to the air ($n = 50$) or water ($n = 50$) method. A Fisher's exact test indicated that the proportions of patients who could complete colonoscopy without sedation in the water group (78%) and the air group (54%) were significantly different. A *t*-test showed that the mean maximum discomfort in the water method group (mean 2.3, SD 1.7) was significantly less than that in the air method group (mean 4.9, SD 2.0).

a) In what circumstances would you use Fisher's exact test? Do you think it was necessary in this study to perform this test to compare the proportions of patients being able to complete colonoscopy without sedation in the water and air method groups? Perform the appropriate calculations to justify your answer. Determine the *P*-value for the comparison of the two proportions.

b) The authors did not explain which kind of *t*-test they performed to compare the mean maximum discomfort in the two groups. Name the *t*-test they would have used. Calculate the *P*-value using this test and the estimated difference in means with a 95% confidence interval.

c) What are the assumptions underlying this test?

d) How important are the assumptions underlying this test? What are the implications if they are not satisfied?

e) Do you think the assumptions underlying the *t*-test are satisfied in this study? Explain your reasoning.

f) How could you test the assumptions if you were given all the data?

g) What alternative test might the authors have used instead of the *t*-test?

Leung J, Mann S, Siao-Salera R, Ransibrahmanakul K, Lim B, Canete W, Samson L, Gutierrez R, Leung FW. A randomized, controlled trial to confirm the beneficial effects of the water method on U.S. veterans undergoing colonoscopy with the option of on-demand sedation. Gastroint Endosc 2010; 73: 103–10.

Envenomation by a *Mesobuthus tamulus* scorpion sting can result in serious cardiovascular effects. Scorpion antivenom is a specific treatment for scorpion sting. Bawasker and Bawasker (2011) designed a randomised clinical trial to assess the efficacy of prazosin combined with scorpion antivenom, compared with prazosin alone, in patients with autonomic storm caused by a scorpion sting. The two variables of primary importance were the time required in hours for recovery after venomous scorpion sting and the percentage of patients achieving complete resolution of the clinical syndrome at the end of 10 hours after administration of the drug treatment. All the patients recovered in this trial.

a) If the hours for recovery are approximately Normally distributed, what test should be used to compare the average time for recovery in the two treatment groups?

b) Using this two-tailed test, how many patients should the investigators have recruited to each equally sized treatment group if they want to detect, with an 80% power at the 5% level of significance, a difference in mean recovery time of at least 4 hours between the two treatments, if they believe the standard deviation of hours for recovery in each group is approximately 6 hours?

c) How would the number of patients in (b) change if the investigators require the power to be 90% instead of 80%?

d) How many patients would the investigators need in each treatment group if they wanted to detect a difference in mean recovery time of 3 hours and all the other requirements remained as those specified in (b)?

e) Suppose the antivenom drug was in short supply and the investigators decide that, instead of having equally sized groups, they want the ratio of the sample sizes to be 2:1, with the larger number in the prazosin alone group. How would they modify their patient numbers in each group using the specifications in (d)?

f) What statistical test should be used to compare, in the two treatment groups, the percentage of patients achieving complete resolution of the clinical syndrome at the end of 10 hours after administration of the drug treatment?

g) Suppose the investigators expected about 20% of the patients in the prazosin group to achieve complete resolution of the clinical syndrome after 10 hours. If they were looking for at least a twofold improvement in the prazosin plus antivenom group, how many patients would they require in each equally sized treatment group, using the two-tailed test named in (f) with an 80% power at a 5% level of significance?

h) If the investigators decided that the specifications in (b) and (g) were optimal, what would be the appropriate sample size of the study?

Bawaskar HS, Bawaskar PH. *Efficacy and safety of scorpion antivenom plus prazosin compared with prazosin alone for venomous scorpion (Mesobuthus tamulus) sting: randomised open label clinical trial. BMJ 2011; 342: c7136.*

Alzheimer's disease is the commonest form of dementia. Cognitive tests aid the diagnosis of dementia and are important in the medical and social management of patients and in the assessment of capacity. The three critical requirements for widespread use by a non-specialist of a cognitive test are that it takes minimal operator time to administer, tests a reasonable range of cognitive functions and is sensitive to mild Alzheimer's disease. Brown *et al.* (2008) designed the TYM ('test your memory') self-administered test to fulfil these requirements. The TYM comprises a series of tasks on which the respondent is scored; the maximum total score is 50, and the score is not influenced by gender. The TYM was evaluated by administering it to 94 patients with mild Alzheimer's disease and 282 age-matched healthy controls. The 'gold standard' diagnosis of Alzheimer's disease was made with the National Institute of Neurological and Communicative Disorders and Stroke and Alzheimer's Disease and Related Disorders Association (NINCDS–ARDRA) criteria for probable Alzheimer's. Using different cut-offs for TYM, the investigators produced a receiver operating characteristic (ROC) curve for TYM scores, differentiating between the controls and patients with mild Alzheimer's disease. The area under the curve was 0.95, and the optimal cut-off for detecting mild Alzheimer's disease was a TYM $\leq$ 42: this gave a sensitivity of 92.5% and a specificity of 86.2%.

a) Explain the meaning of the terms 'sensitivity' and 'specificity'. What do you infer if the sensitivity of the TYM is 92.5% and the specificity is 86.2%?

b) Construct a contingency table showing the number of patients with mild Alzheimer's disease and normal controls with a TYM $\leq$ 42 and > 42.

c) Calculate the positive predictive value (PPV) and negative predictive value (NPV) of the TYM test and interpret them.

d) How is the ROC curve constructed, what does the area under it represent and what can you infer from its value of 0.95?

e) What was the prevalence of mild Alzheimer's disease in this group of individuals? To what extent does the prevalence affect the sensitivity, specificity, PPV and NPV of the TYM test?

f) Why is it not appropriate to use the prevalence determined in (e) as an estimate of the prevalence of mild Alzheimer's disease in the population from which this sample of individuals was taken?

g) What would be the effect on the sensitivity and specificity of raising and of lowering the threshold used to identify individuals likely to have mild Alzheimer's disease?

h) Calculate the likelihood ratio of a positive test result (indicating mild Alzheimer's disease) and interpret its value.

Brown J, Dawson K, Brown LA, Clatworthy P. *Self administered cognitive screening test (TYM) for detection of Alzheimer's disease: cross sectional study. BMJ 2009; 338: b2030.*

A number of scoring systems have been developed to assess the prognosis of those with alcoholic hepatitis. These include the Model of End-Stage Liver Disease (MELD), MELD with sodium (MELD-Na), the Glasgow Alcoholic Hepatitis Score (GAHS), the Lille model and the Age, Bilirubin, International Normalised Ratio and Creatinine (ABIC) score. Sandahl and colleagues (2011) conducted a study to validate and compare the five scores in terms of their ability to predict mortality in an unselected population-based cohort of 274 patients diagnosed with alcoholic hepatitis in Denmark from 1999 to 2008.

Twenty-eight- (16%), 84- (27%) and 180-day (40%) mortality rates were calculated as the proportion of patients who died within 28, 84 and 180 days after hospital admission, respectively. The MELD, MELD-Na, GAHS, Lille and ABIC scores were calculated using information collected at baseline. For each score, the authors calculated the area under the receiver operating characteristic

Table S24.1 AUROC values and measures of performance for the five scoring systems, for assessing 28-, 84- and 180-day mortality. Reproduced with permission of Informa.

	AUROC	Sensitivity	Specificity	Positive predictive value (PPV)	Negative predictive value (NPV)
28-day mortality (16%)					
MELD	0.74	0.69	0.68	0.26	0.93
MELD-Na	0.74	0.90	0.39	0.19	0.96
GAHS	0.75	0.67	0.70	0.27	0.93
Lille	0.78	0.79	0.66	0.27	0.95
ABIC (threshold: 6.71/9)	0.76	0.92/0.44	0.32/0.86	0.18/0.33	0.96/0.90
84-day mortality (27%)					
MELD	0.70	0.63	0.70	0.37	0.87
MELD-Na	0.69	0.81	0.40	0.27	0.89
GAHS	0.72	0.59	0.72	0.37	0.87
Lille	0.77	0.76	0.69	0.41	0.91
ABIC (threshold: 6.71/9)	0.76	0.92/0.37	0.34/0.87	0.28/0.43	0.94/0.83
180-day mortality (40%)					
MELD	0.67	0.60	0.71	0.44	0.82
MELD-Na	0.65	0.76	0.41	0.33	0.82
GAHS	0.69	0.54	0.72	0.43	0.80
Lille	0.75	0.68	0.69	0.46	0.85
ABIC (threshold: 6.71/9)	0.72	0.85/0.35	0.35/0.87	0.33/0.51	0.86/0.77

(AUROC) curve, and the positive and negative predictive values, sensitivity and specificity using cut-offs from the original study publications (MELD-Na: 21; GAHS: 9; Lille: 0.45 and ABIC: 6.71 and 9) or from subsequent publications (MELD: 21). Table S24.1 shows the performance characteristics of the five scores for 28-, 84- and 180-day mortality using these cut-off values.

a) What feature of model performance does the AUROC measure? How is the AUROC calculated, and how do you interpret the value for the Lille score shown in Table S24.1 for 28-day mortality?

b) How do the five scores compare in terms of AUROC, and how do the AUROC values change as the period over which mortality is measured lengthens?

c) Describe how the authors would have calculated the sensitivity, specificity, PPV and NPV for the MELD score at 84 days.

d) Describe the differences seen in sensitivity, specificity, PPV and NPV for the five scores when assessing 84-day mortality. How do these measures of model performance change as the period over which mortality is measured lengthens from 28 days to 180 days? Comment on the possible clinical implications of these changes.

e) Why do you think the PPV values are so low for all scores, whereas the NPV values are much higher? Why do you think the measures of all model performance change in this way as the period over which mortality is measured lengthens?

Sandahl TD, Jepsen P, Ott P, Vilstrup H. Validation of prognostic scores for clinical use in patients with alcoholic hepatitis. Scand J Gastroenterol 2011; 46(9): 1127–32.

S25

Progression to end-stage liver disease is an important cause of mortality and morbidity in individuals infected with HIV. Diagnosis of end-stage liver disease, however, generally requires a liver biopsy, which is invasive and often painful. Thus, several non-invasive scores have been proposed that aim to identify patients with liver fibrosis. These include the FIB-4 score (a score based on the patient's age, aspartate

Table S25.1 Number (%) of patients with Classes 1, 2 and 3 liver failure, classified according to FIB-4 and APRI scores. Reproduced with permission of Oxford University Press.

APRI	FIB-4, *n* (%) patients		
	Class 1	Class 2	Class 3
Class 1	**718 (64.6)**	66 (5.9)	1 (0.1)
Class 2	110 (9.9)	**164 (14.7)**	20 (1.8)
Class 3	4 (0.4)	12 (1.1)	**17 (1.5)**

aminotransferase (AST) and alanine aminotransferase (ALT) levels and platelet count) and the AST-to-Platelet Ratio Index (APRI) (which is based on the patient's AST level and platelet count only). Although the APRI score has been validated in those with HIV and hepatitis C virus infection, no formal validation exists in those infected with HIV alone. Thus, Mendeni and colleagues (2011) assessed the concordance of these two scores for the staging of liver fibrosis in individuals infected with HIV with no evidence of hepatitis C or B virus co-infection. The authors calculated APRI and FIB-4 scores on 1112 mono-infected individuals from the Hepatotoxicity of Different Kinds of Antiretrovirals Study, which followed individuals to study liver complications after individuals started combination antiretroviral therapy (cART). Individuals were classified as having Class 1, 2 or 3 liver failure if their APRI (FIB-4) scores were ≤0.5 (≤1.45), 0.51 to 1.5 (1.46 to 3.25) or >3.25 (>1.5), respectively. The classifications of patients based on the two scores are shown in Table S25.1.

a) Calculate and interpret the kappa coefficient for the data shown in Table S25.1. What modification of kappa might also be used in this situation and why?

b) Comment on the use of the kappa coefficient to determine the reliability of either score for identifying those with liver failure. If this was a primary aim of the study, what approach might the authors have used?

c) Had the authors combined Classes 2 and 3 for the purposes of calculating kappa, what would have been the effect on their assessment of agreement between the scores? Why is this?

Mendeni M, Foca E, Gotti D, Ladisa N, Angarano G, Albini L, Castelnuovo F, Carosi G, Quiros-Roldan E, Torti C. Evaluation of liver fibrosis: concordance analysis between noninvasive scores (APRI and FIB-4) evolution and predictors in a cohort of HIV-infected patients without hepatitis C and B infection. Clin Infect Dis 2011; 52: 1164–73.

S26

Limitations in physical activity and fatigue are acknowledged as key problems in multiple sclerosis (MS), with up to 85% of patients reporting walking difficulties. Specifying these problems has great importance for understanding their impact on activities of daily living. A central issue in this process is to gather objective information regarding the real quantity and type of daily activities performed in the patient's own home environment, recognising that obtaining information on only one occasion may be unreliable. Ambulatory monitoring (AM) is a system that uses accelerometers attached to the trunk and legs and allows the collection of information about the type, amount and pattern of mobility-related activities. Rieberg *et al.* (2010) assessed the repeatability of 24-hour monitoring of mobility-related activities in 43 ambulatory patients with MS. The AM was applied and removed in the participant's own home by a trained research assistant. Twenty-four-hour monitoring was performed twice, with an interval of exactly 1 week between the two assessments, assuming that activity patterns remained approximately the same between similar weekdays. Amongst other measures, data were collected on the number of hours that each participant walked in each of the two 24-hour assessments. The mean of the difference in hours walked between the two assessments was −0.01 hours, and the standard deviation (SD) of the differences was 0.50 hours. A Bland and Altman diagram was constructed, as shown in Figure S26.1.

a) Do you believe there is a systematic difference in the hours walked between the two assessments? Perform a relevant hypothesis test to investigate this.

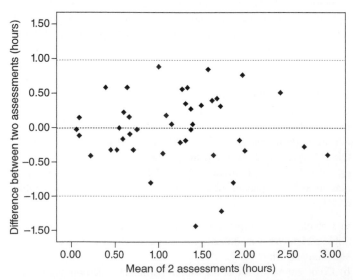

Figure S26.1 Bland and Altman diagram assessing the repeatability of ambulatory monitoring in patients with multiple sclerosis. Reproduced with permission of Elsevier.

b) Calculate the limits of agreement in the Bland and Altman diagram and interpret them.
c) Is it sensible to calculate a single measure of repeatability? Explain your answer.
d) Calculate the British Standards Institution repeatability coefficient and explain what it represents.
e) Do you believe that the 24-hour ambulatory monitoring of hours walked in ambulatory patients with MS was repeatable?
f) Explain why it would be inappropriate to calculate the Pearson correlation coefficient between the first and second assessments of hours walked as a measure of repeatability.
g) What measure would provide an appropriate index of reliability? What value does it take if there is perfect agreement between the repeated observations?

Rietberg MB, van Wegen EE, Uitdehaag BM, de Vet HC, Kwakkel G. How reproducible is home-based 24-hour ambulatory monitoring of motor activity in patients with multiple sclerosis? Arch Phys Med Rehabil 2010; 91: 1537–41.

S27

Polyzos *et al.* (2010) were interested in determining whether treatment of periodontal disease during pregnancy is associated with a reduction in the number of preterm births (<37 weeks) among all successful pregnancies. They identified a total of 11 randomised controlled clinical trials, each comparing treatment with scaling and root planing to no treatment. Initially the authors calculated the odds ratio of preterm birth in the treatment group compared to the control group in each study, and then performed a meta-analysis, combining the results from the different studies. Methodological quality of the studies was assessed with Cochrane's risk of bias tool: five trials were considered to be of high quality and six of low quality. The forest plot in Figure S27.1 shows results for the 11 studies together and separately for the high- and low-quality studies. Figure S27.2 is a funnel plot of the results.

a) Define the null hypothesis for a test of heterogeneity in a meta-analysis and explain what I^2 represents.
b) Explain why a separate meta-analysis for the high- and low-quality studies is recommended.
c) Explain why a fixed-effect analysis was used for the high- and low-quality studies.
d) Why are the boxes, representing the estimated odds ratios in the different studies, of varying sizes?
e) Interpret the overall odds ratios for the high- and low-quality studies separately.
f) What conclusion do you draw about using scaling and root planing to treat periodontal disease in pregnancy to reduce the preterm birth rate?
g) What do you think the effect estimate on the horizontal axis of the funnel plot represents?
h) What do you infer from the funnel plot? Do you think your interpretation of the results from the funnel plot would affect the overall conclusion about using scaling and root planing to treat periodontal disease in pregnancy to reduce the preterm birth rate? Explain both answers.

Polyzos NP, Polyzos IP, Zavos A, Valachis A, Mauri D, Papanikolaou EG, Tzioras S, Messinis IE. Obstetric outcomes after treatment of periodontal disease during pregnancy: systematic review and meta-analysis. BMJ 2010; 341: c7017.

Study or subgroup	Treatment Events/total	No Treatment Events/total	Odds ratio (M-H, fixed) (95% confidence interval)	Weight (%)	Odds ratio (M-H, fixed) (95% CI)
Low-quality trials					
Lopez (2002)	7/168	14/190		4.2	0.55 (0.22 to 1.39)
Lopez (2005)	18/563	17/282		7.3	0.51 (0.26 to 1.02)
Sadatmansuri (2006)	0/15	3/15		1.1	0.12 (0.01 to 2.45)
Offenbacher (2006)	9/35	14/32		3.6	0.45 (0.16 to 1.25)
Tarranum (2007)	53/99	68/89		11.1	0.36 (0.19 to 0.67)
Oliveira (2007)	27/116	31/117		7.9	0.84 (0.46 to 1.53)
Subtotal (95% CI)	114/996	147/725		35.2	0.52 (0.38 to 0.72)
Test for heterogeneity: $\chi^2 = 4.95$, df = 5, $P = 0.42$, $I^2 = 0\%$					
Test for overall effect: $z = 4.01$, $P<0.001$					
High-quality trials					
Jeffcoat (2003)	5/123	11/123		3.5	0.43 (0.15 to 1.28)
Michalowicz (2006)	44/402	38/391		11.4	1.14 (0.72 to 1.81)
Offenbacher (2009)	91/881	73/880		21.8	1.27 (0.92 to 1.76)
Newnham (2009)	52/538	50/535		15.1	1.04 (0.69 to 1.56)
Macones (2010)	58/359	47/361		13.1	1.29 (0.85 to 1.95)
Subtotal (95% CI)	250/2303	219/2290		64.8	1.15 (0.95 to 1.40)
Test for heterogeneity: $\chi^2 = 4.02$, df = 4, $P = 0.40$, $I^2 = 1\%$					
Test for overall effect: $z = 1.45$, $P = 0.15$					
Total (95% CI)	364/3299	366/3015		100.0	0.93 (0.79 to 1.10)
Test for heterogeneity: $\chi^2 = 25.94$, df = 10, $P = 0.004$, $I^2 = 61\%$					
Test for overall effect: $z = 0.86$, $P = 0.39$					

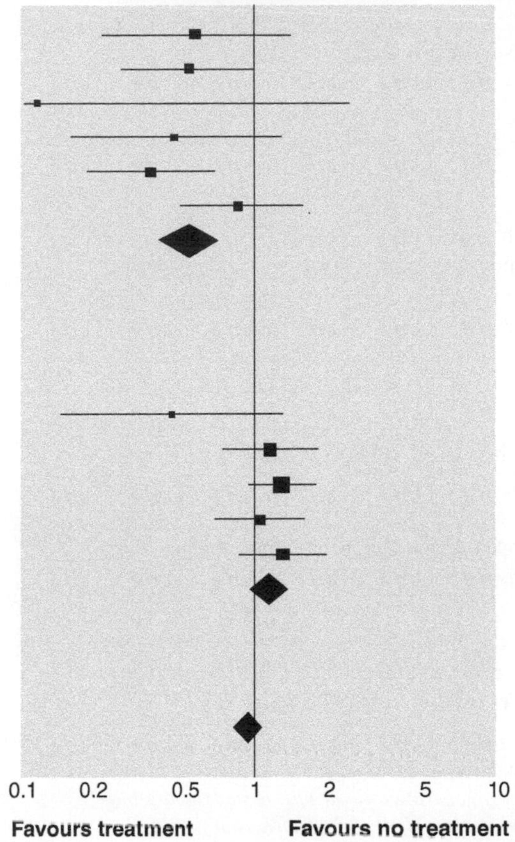

0.1 0.2 0.5 1 2 5 10

Favours treatment   Favours no treatment

Figure S27.1 Forest plot from a meta-analysis of studies assessing the effect of periodontal treatment during pregnancy on preterm birth. Reproduced with permission of BMJ Publishing Group Ltd.

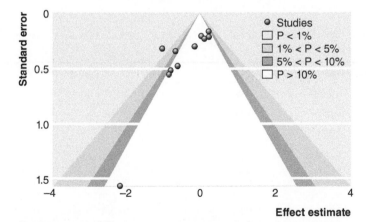

Figure S27.2 Funnel plot from a meta-analysis of studies assessing the effect of periodontal treatment during pregnancy on preterm birth. Reproduced with permission of BMJ Publishing Group Ltd.

S28

Thourani and colleagues (2011) conducted a study to investigate the short-term and long-term outcomes of patients with end-stage renal disease who were receiving dialysis and who underwent cardiac valve surgery. In particular, they were interested in investigating the impact of the type of valve (biological or mechanical) on outcomes among patients who underwent isolated aortic or mitral valve prosthesis. The primary outcomes examined were in-hospital mortality, major adverse cardiac events (MACE – a composite outcome of death, permanent stroke and myocardial infarction) and long-term mortality. Follow-up on those patients who remained alive on 31 December 2007 was right-censored. Data were 100% complete for each valve surgery type, valve implant type and all major postoperative hospital outcomes. However, data were missing on race (6.6% of patients), ejection fraction (18.0%), New York Heart classification (19.9%), last creatinine level (12.8%) and predicted risk of mortality (37.4%). Therefore, the authors used a multiple imputation algorithm to impute the missing values. The authors used Kaplan–Meier curves to demonstrate postoperative survival in strata defined by valve location and type, and compared outcomes in these strata using the log-rank test.

In total, 149 individuals were included in the study, 100 who underwent an isolated aortic valve replacement and 49 who underwent an isolated mitral valve replacement. Ninety-nine individuals received a biological valve (BIO), and 50 received a mechanical valve (MECH). Patients receiving a biological valve were generally at higher preoperative risk, were older and were more likely to be male, be of Caucasian race, have diabetes, be smokers and have urgent-emergent status. Long-term survival rates stratified by valve location and type are shown in Figure S28.1, with information on other postoperative complications shown in Table S28.1. In univariable analysis, median survival did not differ by implant type, either overall ($P = 0.87$) or stratified by valve location (aortic valve: $P = 0.83$; mitral valve: $P = 0.79$). After adjustment for potential confounders using a Cox regression analysis, the estimate of the effect of a biological valve was protective but not statistically significant (overall: hazard ratio = 0.73 (95% confidence interval 0.48, 1.10), $P = 0.13$; aortic valve: 0.82 (0.45, 1.53), $P = 0.54$ and mitral valve: 0.68 (0.24, 1.93), $P = 0.47$).

a) Using Figure S28.1a, b, read off the median survival times among individuals undergoing an isolated aortic valve replacement and an isolated mitral valve replacement (for the biological and mechanical valves separately). Comment on the reliability of these estimates.

b) Comment on the authors' conclusion that there was no overall effect of the type of valve on survival (i.e. ignoring location). Is there any evidence that the impact of valve type varies by the valve location? What test should the authors perform to formally assess this?

c) Prolonged ventilation appears to be more common among those undergoing a mitral valve replacement with a biological valve. Comment on this finding.

d) Why did the authors use methods (multiple imputation) to impute the missing values for race, ejection fraction, New York Heart Classification, last creatinine level and predicted risk of mortality?

Thourani VH, Sarin EL, Keeling B, Kilgo PD, Guyton RA, Dara AB, Puskas JD, Chen EP, Cooper WA, Vega JD, Morris CD, Lattouf OM. Long-term survival for patients with preoperative renal failure undergoing bioprosthetic or mechanical valve replacement. Ann Thorac Surg 2011; 91: 1127–34.

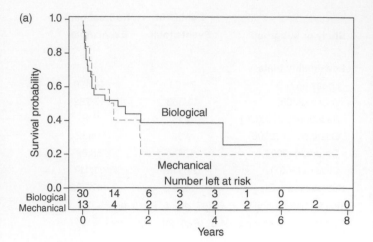

(a)

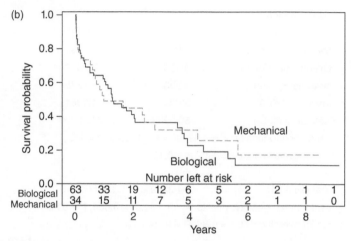

(b)

Figure S28.1 Kaplan–Meier survival estimates stratified by type of valve received (biological or mechanical). (a) Isolated aortic valve replacements and (b) isolated mitral valve replacements. Reproduced with permission of Elsevier.

Table S28.1 Postoperative complications by valve location and valve type (values shown are n (%) unless otherwise stated). Reproduced with permission of Elsevier.

Complication		Isolated aortic valve replacement			Isolated mitral valve replacement		
	Type of valve	BIO ($n = 65$)	MECH ($n = 35$)	P-value	BIO ($n = 34$)	MECH ($n = 15$)	P-value
Myocardial infarction		0 (0.0)	0 (0.0)	1.00	0 (0.0)	0 (0.0)	1.00
Stroke		2 (3.1)	1 (2.9)	0.95	2 (5.9)	1 (6.7)	0.92
Mediastinitis		2 (3.1)	3 (8.6)	0.23	0 (0.0)	1 (6.7)	0.13
Worsening renal failure		3 (4.6)	0 (0.0)	0.20	2 (5.9)	1 (6.7)	0.92
Septicaemia		8 (12.3)	3 (8.6)	0.57	6 (17.7)	2 (13.3)	0.71
Heart block requiring pacemaker		0 (0.0)	2 (5.7)	0.05	1 (2.9)	2 (13.3)	0.16
Multi-system organ failure		5 (7.7)	2 (5.7)	0.71	4 (11.8)	1 (6.7)	0.59
Re-exploration for haemorrhage		6 (9.2)	3 (8.6)	0.91	3 (8.8)	0 (0.0)	0.24
Postoperative pneumonia		9 (13.9)	1 (2.9)	0.08	5 (14.7)	2 (13.3)	0.90
Postoperative ventilator hours (mean ± standard deviation (SD))		102 ± 182	48 ± 83	0.05	142 ± 231	133 ± 411	0.94
Prolonged ventilation		22 (33.9)	7 (20.0)	0.15	23 (67.7)	3 (20.0)	0.002
Postoperative intra-aortic balloon counterpulsation insertion		0 (0.0)	0 (0.0)	1.00	0 (0.0)	0 (0.0)	1.00
Gastrointestinal complication		8 (12.3)	3 (8.6)	0.57	8 (23.5)	1 (6.7)	0.16
Total intensive care unit length of stay (hours) (mean ± SD)		198 ± 255	144 ± 162	0.42	214 ± 244	353 ± 673	0.67
Postoperative length of stay (days) (mean ± SD)		12.9 ± 13.1	12.7 ± 10.6	0.93	16.3 ± 11.5	27.1 ± 27.7	0.17
In-hospital mortality		11 (16.9)	6 (17.1)	0.98	8 (23.5)	4 (26.7)	0.81
Observed or expected mortality		1.03	1.32	–	1.10	2.20	–

There are concerns that medical staff fatigue may increase the risk of medical errors, with several studies showing that night-time medical care is associated with worse clinical outcomes. George and colleagues (2011) used data from the United Network for Organ Sharing (UNOS) transplant database to investigate whether performing orthotopic heart transplants or lung transplants at night was associated with adverse outcomes for transplant recipients. The data set included all adults older than 18 years who underwent heart or lung transplant from January 2000 to June 2010. The primary endpoint of the study was all-cause mortality. Patients were grouped according to the time of day of their operation, with daytime being defined as between 7 AM to 7 PM, and night-time from 7 PM to 7 AM. The association between operative time of day (as a binary covariate) and survival was described using Kaplan–Meier curves with the authors focusing on 30-day, 90-day and 1-year survival rates. Cox proportional hazards regression models were used to assess the independent associations of operative time of day with survival at the three time points, after adjusting for potential confounding factors. Potential confounding factors were identified as those that were supported by previously published literature, biological plausibility or a P-value <0.2 from univariable analyses. These potential confounding factors were selected for inclusion in the final model using a forwards and backwards stepwise selection process.

The final data set included information on 27 118 patients undergoing transplant. Of the 16 573 heart transplants, 8346 (50.4%) were undertaken during the day, and 8227 (49.6%) during the night. Of the 10 545 lung transplants, 5179 (49.1%) were undertaken during the day, and 5366 (50.9%) during the night. Over a median follow-up of 32.2 months, 8061 (29.0%) patients died. There were several differences between patients who underwent transplant during daytime and night-time. In particular, those undergoing heart transplant during the day had higher creatinine levels, lower mean pulmonary artery pressures, lower pulmonary capillary wedge pressures, more preoperative dependence on inotropes and less preoperative ventricular assist device implantation; furthermore, the donors of these patients were younger, had less hypertension and more commonly needed inotropic support before organ recovery. Among those undergoing lung transplant, those receiving transplants during the day were less likely to be older, more likely to be white, less likely to have a diagnosis of idiopathic pulmonary fibrosis, had a higher forced vital capacity, were less likely to be hospitalised or in the ICU preoperatively, were more likely to have donors with a smoking history and tended to have a longer time on the waiting list prior to transplant.

Survival rates (%) at 30 days, 90 days and 1 year (from Kaplan–Meier plots) are shown in Table S29.1, along with the P-values from log-rank tests.

a) Why did the authors choose to use Kaplan–Meier methods and Cox proportional hazards regression models to analyse this data set? What alternative appropriate approach could have been used? Why would a logistic regression model *not* be appropriate in this situation?

b) The authors report that the median follow-up time of patients in the study was 32.2 months – why did they report the median follow-up time rather than the mean follow-up time?

c) Interpret the results of the analysis of lung transplant outcomes, particularly focusing on the finding at 90 days. What is your view about this finding?

d) What are the differences between the P-values shown in column 4 and those in column 6 of Table S29.1?

e) What is the main assumption of the Cox proportional hazards regression model? Do the results of the study provide any evidence that this assumption may not be valid? Give reasons for your answer.

f) The authors selected potential confounding variables for inclusion in the final model on the basis of a forwards and backwards selection process. What does this process entail? Why did the authors take this approach? What are its limitations?

g) Calculate the number needed to treat with heart transplants during the daytime to prevent one death within 90 days? Interpret and comment on this value.

George TJ, Arnaoutakis GJ, Merlo CA, Kemp CD, Baumgartner WA, Conte JV, Shah AS. Association of operative time of day with outcomes after thoracic organ transplant. JAMA 2011; 305: 2193–9.

Table S29.1 30-day, 90-day and 1-year survival rates (%) among individuals undergoing heart and lung transplants

	Time of day of surgery		P-value (log-rank)	Adjusted relative hazard (night vs. day)* (95% CI)	P-value*
	Daytime	Night-time			
	% (95% confidence interval (CI))	% (95% CI)			
Heart transplants					
30-day survival	95.0 (94.5, 95.5)	95.2 (94.7, 95.7)	0.78	1.05 (0.83, 1.32)	0.67
90-day survival	92.6 (92.0, 93.1)	92.7 (92.1, 93.3)	0.93	1.05 (0.88, 1.26)	0.59
1-year survival	88.0 (87.2, 88.7)	87.7 (86.9, 88.4)	0.46	1.05 (0.91, 1.21)	0.47
Lung transplants					
30-day survival	96.0 (95.4, 96.5)	95.5 (94.9, 96.1)	0.13	1.22 (0.97, 1.55)	0.09
90-day survival	92.7 (91.9, 93.4)	91.7 (90.9, 92.4)	0.03	1.23 (1.04, 1.47)	0.02
1-year survival	83.8 (82.8, 84.9)	82.6 (81.5, 83.6)	0.08	1.08 (0.96, 1.22)	0.19

*Relative hazards and P-values obtained from multivariable Cox proportional hazards regression model with adjustment for differences in donor and recipient status at time of transplant.

Part 3: Critical appraisal
Randomised controlled trial: template

The following template, based on the CONSORT statement (www.consort-statement.org), can be used to critically appraise and evaluate the evidence in published papers reporting a randomised controlled trial (RCT).

A. Title and abstract
1. Is the trial identified as a RCT in the title?
2. Does the abstract summarise the trial's primary objective, design, methods, results and conclusions?

B. Introduction
1. Is a proper description provided of the scientific background, and is the rationale for the trial explained sufficiently? Has all the relevant information from previous studies and other available evidence been included?
2. Is the primary aim of the trial indicated, preferably in relation to a relevant hypothesis based on the outcome of interest, and are secondary objectives described?

C. Methods
1. **Trial design** Is the trial design described adequately? Are any aspects of the design utilised to avoid bias fully described? For example:
   a) *Randomisation.* Are full details of the randomisation process provided, including the method used to generate the random allocation sequence, the type of randomisation, steps taken to conceal the allocation sequence and details of the implementation of the randomisation (e.g. who enrolled the participants and who assigned the participants to the interventions)?
   b) *Blinding.* To what extent was the study blind? If relevant, is a description provided of the similarity of the interventions?
   c) *Allocation concealment.* Was the allocation sequence concealed from the staff who recruited patients for the trial?
2. **Participants**
   a) Is there a complete description of the eligibility (inclusion and exclusion) criteria for the participants?
   b) Was the study conducted using an appropriate spectrum of patients?
3. **Interventions**
   a) Is the intervention (treatment and/or placebo, if appropriate) for each group described in sufficient detail?
   b) Were the groups treated in similar fashion, aside from the fact that they received different interventions?
4. **Outcomes**
   a) Is consideration given to all the important outcomes?
   b) Are the primary and secondary outcomes defined precisely?
   c) Were there any changes to the outcomes after the trial started?
5. **Sample size**
   a) Is there a power statement to justify the overall sample size? Does this power statement indicate the form of the statistical analysis on which it is based, and does it include a specification of the values of all the factors that affect sample size for this calculation?
   b) If relevant, is there a full explanation of any interim analysis, including the steps taken to reduce the Type I error rate?
   c) If subgroup analyses have been performed, is there a justification for the subgroup sample sizes, based on power calculations, and a description of the steps taken to reduce the Type I error rate? Alternatively, are these subgroup analyses specified as being *exploratory* in nature, with an indication that they may be under-powered?
6. **Statistical methods**
   a) Are all the statistical methods used to compare groups for primary and secondary outcomes identified?
   b) Are the statistical methods appropriate (e.g. have underlying assumptions been verified, and have dependencies in the data (e.g. pairing) been taken into account in the analysis?)?
   c) Is there a description of additional analyses, such as subgroup analyses? Were any additional analyses undertaken specified *a priori*, or were they *post hoc* analyses?

D. Results
1. **Participant numbers and dates**
   a) Is there a full explanation (preferably in a participant flow chart), for each treatment group, of the numbers of participants who were randomly assigned, received the intended treatment and were analysed for the primary outcome?
   b) If relevant, are numbers of and reasons for losses to follow-up and exclusions after randomisation documented?
   c) Are dates provided which define the periods of recruitment and follow-up?

Medical Statistics at a Glance Workbook, First Edition. Aviva Petrie and Caroline Sabin.

2. **Baseline data**
   a) Is there a table which shows the baseline demographic and clinical characteristics for each group?
   b) Are the groups comparable?
3. **Numbers analysed**
   a) Is there a specification of whether an 'intention-to-treat' (ITT) analysis was performed? Is a justification given for the choice of analysis (ITT or other), and is this appropriate?
   b) If there were protocol deviations, was a sensitivity analysis performed (e.g. as per protocol analysis or an analysis with imputed data for missing observations)?
4. **Outcomes of interest**
   a) *Main outcome of interest.* Is an appropriate summary measure given for the main outcome variable (i.e. that which relates to the primary aim of the study) for each comparison group? An example is the rate, risk or odds of occurrence of the outcome (e.g. death) if the outcome variable is *binary*, stating results in absolute numbers when feasible; or the mean (median) if the outcome variable is *numerical*.
   b) *Magnitude of the effect of interest.* Is there an indication of the magnitude of the effect of interest? Examples include a ratio such as the relative rate, risk or odds, or a difference such as the absolute difference in risk, if the outcome variable is *binary*; or a difference in means (medians) if the main outcome variable is *numerical*.
   c) *Precision of the effect of interest.* Is there an indication of the precision of the effect of interest (e.g. a 95% confidence interval or standard error)?
5. **Additional analyses** If additional (e.g. subgroup) analyses were performed, are their results provided, and are any exploratory analyses distinguished from those that were pre-specified?
6. **Harms** Are all important harms in each group documented?

E. Discussion

1. **Deciding whether the results are important**
   a) Are the key findings summarised with reference to the trial objectives?
   b) Do the results make **biological sense**? If a **confidence interval** for the effect of interest (e.g. the difference in treatment means) has been provided:
      (i) Would you regard the observed effect clinically important (irrespective of whether or not the result of the relevant hypothesis test is statistically significant) if the lower limit of the confidence interval represented the true value of the effect?
      (ii) Would you regard the observed effect clinically important if the upper limit of the confidence interval represented the true value of the effect?
      (iii) Are your answers to questions (i) and (ii) sufficiently similar to declare the results of the study unambiguous and important?
   c) Is there an evaluation of the **number of patients needed to treat** (NNT) with the experimental treatment rather than the control treatment in order to prevent one of them from developing the 'bad' outcome?
2. **Limitations** Is there a discussion of all the trial limitations, including sources of potential bias and imprecision?
3. **Generalisability** Is there a discussion of the generalisability (external validity) of the trial findings (i.e. the extent to which the participants are representative of the wider population)?
4. **Interpretation** Taking the benefits and harms into consideration, as well as the limitations of the trial, any multiple testing and subgroup analyses, is the interpretation of the trial findings consistent with the results?

F. Other information

1. **Registration** Are the trial registration number and the name of the trial registry provided?
2. **Protocol** Is there information about where the protocol can be accessed?
3. **Funding** Are sources of funding documented?
4. **Conflict of interest** Is there a conflict of interest statement for each of the investigators?

Randomised controlled trial: Paper 1

The following paper is from *Obstetrics & Gynecology* 2003; 102(6): 1250–4. Reproduced with permission from Elsevier.

A Randomized, Placebo-Controlled Trial of Corticosteroids for Hyperemesis Due to Pregnancy

Nicole P. Yost, MD, Donald D. McIntire, PhD, Frank H. Wians Jr, PhD, Susan M. Ramin, MD, Jody A. Balko, and Kenneth J. Leveno, MD

OBJECTIVE: Hyperemesis gravidarum, a severe form of nausea and vomiting due to pregnancy for which there is no proven pharmacological treatment, is the third leading cause for hospitalization during pregnancy. Corticosteroids are commonly used for the treatment of nausea and vomiting due to cancer chemotherapy–induced emesis and might prove useful in hyperemesis gravidarum.

METHODS: A randomized, double-blind, placebo-controlled trial was conducted in 126 women who previously had not responded to outpatient therapy for hyperemesis gravidarum during the first half of pregnancy. Intravenous methylprednisolone (125 mg) was followed by an oral prednisone taper (40 mg for 1 day, 20 mg for 3 days, 10 mg for 3 days, 5 mg for 7 days) versus an identical-appearing placebo regimen. All women also received promethazine 25 mg and metoclopramide 10 mg intravenously every 6 hours for 24 hours, followed by the same regimen administered orally as needed until discharge. The primary study outcome was the number of women requiring rehospitalization for hyperemesis gravidarum.

RESULTS: A total of 110 women delivered at our hospital and had pregnancy outcomes available for analysis; 56 were randomized to corticosteroids and 54 were administered placebo. Nineteen women in each study group required rehospitalization (34% versus 35%, $P = .89$, for corticosteroids versus placebo, respectively).

CONCLUSION: The addition of parenteral and oral corticosteroids to the treatment of women with hyperemesis gravidarum did not reduce the need for rehospitalization later in pregnancy. (Obstet Gynecol 2003;102:1250–4. © 2003 by The American College of Obstetricians and Gynecologists.)

Nausea and vomiting are the most common symptoms experienced in early pregnancy and affect 50% to 80% of women.[1] One to 3% of these women experience hyperemesis gravidarum, a severe form of vomiting due to pregnancy characterized by weight loss, electrolyte abnormalities, dehydration, and ketonuria.[1] Severe nausea and vomiting is the third leading cause for hospitalization during pregnancy,[2] with a financial burden on the American health system estimated at $130 million per year.[1] It is estimated that 206 hours are lost from paid work for each woman who has nausea and vomiting during early pregnancy.[3] Complications, albeit uncommon, associated with hyperemesis gravidarum include Wernicke,[5] encephalopathy,[4] rhabdomyolysis,[5] coagulopathy,[6] and low birth weight infants.[7]

In 1959, Geiger and et al,[8] in a double-blind, placebo-controlled trial, showed that Bendectin aided in the treatment of nausea and vomiting of pregnancy. Bendectin became the first pharmaceutical option designated specifically for controlling symptoms of nausea and vomiting due to pregnancy, but it was removed from the market in 1983 because of claims of teratogenicity, which were subsequently proven to be unsubstantiated.[9] Since then, there have been few randomized trials to assess different treatment modalities. Corticosteroids have been proposed to modify the chemoreceptor trigger zone in the brain[10] that is responsible for nausea and vomiting, and on this basis, corticosteroids have been used successfully for many years to treat cancer chemotherapy–induced emesis.[11,12] Our goal was to estimate the effect of corticosteroids in reducing the number of women requiring rehospitalization for hyperemesis gravidarum as has been described in one randomized trial.[13]

MATERIALS AND METHODS

From July 6, 1998, to August 22, 2001, all women presenting to Parkland Memorial Hospital, Dallas, complaining of nausea and vomiting during the first half of pregnancy (less than 20 weeks' gestation) were asked to participate in a study of the efficacy of intravenous methylprednisolone and oral prednisone. Women considered eligible for this study were those who previously had not responded to outpatient therapy and who dem-

From the University of Texas Southwestern Medical Center, Department of Obstetrics and Gynecology, and Department of Pathology, Dallas, Texas and the University of Texas Houston Medical School, Department of Obstetrics and Gynecology, Houston, Texas.

1250

onstrated 3+ or 4+ dipstick urinary ketones as evidence of severe dehydration. Outpatient therapy for hyperemesis is standardized at our hospital and consists of promethazine 25 mg every 6 hours as needed. Before enrollment into the study, an ultrasound was performed to exclude molar pregnancy, to confirm a live fetus, and to establish gestational age. The study protocol was approved by the Institutional Review Board of the University of Texas Southwestern Medical Center, and informed written consent was obtained from all the women. Staffing of the obstetric service is provided by faculty from the Department of Obstetrics and Gynecology at the University of Texas Southwestern Medical School.

The women enrolled in the study were all provided the prevailing treatment for persistent hyperemesis gravidarum at our hospital. This treatment included admission and intravenous hydration with crystalloid until ketonuria cleared. The first liter of crystalloid included thiamine 100 mg. Conventional treatment also included promethazine 25 mg and metoclopramide 10 mg intravenously every 6 hours for 24 hours, followed by the same regimen administered as needed orally until discharge from the hospital. The women were also randomly administered, in a double-blind fashion, methylprednisolone 125 mg intravenously or placebo. This was followed by a tapering regimen of oral prednisone or an identical-appearing placebo (40 mg for 1 day, 20 mg for 3 days, 10 mg for 3 days, and 5 mg for 7 days). These study drugs were dispensed by the Investigational Drug Service of Parkland Hospital. Randomization was performed by computer-generated blocks of 20.

Women with persistent vomiting on day 2 of hospitalization and randomized to methylprednisolone received an additional 80-mg dose, and similar women in the placebo arm received an identical-appearing placebo drug. The decision to give an additional dose of study drug was made exclusively by the principal investigator (NY). Both groups of women were provided crackers and juice upon request and were advanced to a regular diet as tolerated, at which time discharge was permitted. Each woman was counseled by a nutritionist before discharge. At discharge, all women also received promethazine 25 mg every 6 hours as needed and metoclopramide 10 mg every 6 hours as needed in addition to their oral study drug taper. This treatment approach was also used in women requiring readmission for hyperemesis gravidarum. Study drug assignment during subsequent admissions was identical to that used for the initial admission; there were no crossovers.

All women enrolled into this trial routinely underwent a battery of laboratory tests to include assessments of

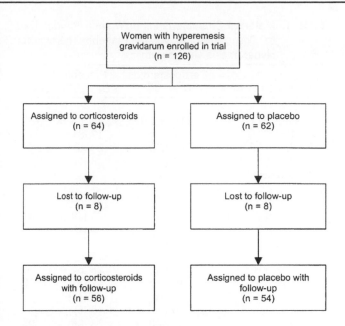

Figure 1. Summary of patients randomized to corticosteroids or placebo treatment.

Yost. Steroids for Hyperemesis. Obstet Gynecol 2003.

thyroid function, liver function, pancreas (amylase and lipase), electrolytes, and human chorionic gonadotropin.

A minimum sample size of 70 women was estimated to be necessary, assuming that corticosteroid therapy would reduce the number of women requiring rehospitalization from 30% to 5%. This assumption was based on a published report that suggested corticosteroids virtually eliminated the need for rehospitalization.[13] This sample size provided a power of 80% for a two-sided test with a significance of error rate .05.

Statistical analysis included χ^2, Student t test, and Wilcoxon signed-rank test. $P < .05$ was considered statistically significant. Analysis was performed by SAS 8.2 (SAS Institute, Cary, NC).

RESULTS

A total of 126 women were enrolled into this trial, and 110 women (87%) were subsequently delivered at Parkland Hospital (Figure 1). The remainder were lost to follow-up. The 16 excluded women were not significantly different from the remainder of the cohort with respect to maternal characteristics, laboratory tests, and course before randomization. The results were analyzed on an intent-to-treat basis using the 56 women with follow-up and randomized to corticosteroid therapy compared with the 54 women administered placebo. The characteristics of the women in these two study groups were similar (Table 1). The mean gestational age

Table 1. Maternal Characteristics in Women Randomized to Corticosteroids Versus Placebo Therapy for Hyperemesis Gravidarum

Characteristic	Corticosteroids (n = 56)	Placebo (n = 54)	P value
Age (y)			
Mean ± SD	22.9 ± 4.9	22.3 ± 4.6	.50
16–19	12 (21)	17 (31)	.39
20–30	41 (73)	33 (61)	
31–34	1 (2)	3 (6)	
35 or older	2 (4)	1 (2)	
Race			
Hispanic	32 (57)	31 (57)	
African American	21 (38)	21 (39)	.51
White	1 (2)	2 (4)	
Other	2 (4)	0	
Parity			
Nulliparous	27 (48)	28 (52)	
Para 1	16 (29)	17 (31)	.80
Para 2	10 (18)	6 (11)	
Para 3	3 (5)	3 (6)	
Singleton	55 (98)	53 (98)	.98
Prior preterm birth	2 (4)	3 (6)	.62
Gestational age at randomization (wk), mean ± SD	11.0 ± 2.7	10.8 ± 2.7	.69

Unless otherwise indicated, all data are presented as n (%).

at randomization was 11.0 ± 2.7 weeks in women administered corticosteroids compared with 10.8 ± 2.7 (P = .69) in women who received placebo. Shown in Table 2 are laboratory results at randomization for women according to study drug assignment. There were no significant differences. The disease course before and after randomization was not different between the two study groups (Table 3). Of the 19 women in each group

Table 2. Laboratory Characteristics in Women with Hyperemesis Gravidarum and Randomized to Corticosteroids or Placebo

Characteristic	Corticosteroids (n = 56)	Placebo (n = 54)	P value
Thyroid function			
Low TSH	31 (55)	27 (50)	.57
Liver function			
Elevated bilirubin	8 (14)	10 (19)	.55
Elevated AST or ALT	12 (21)	11 (20)	.89
Pancreas			
Elevated amylase	4 (7)	6 (11)	.47
Elevated lipase	10 (18)	10 (19)	.93
Creatinine >0.9 mg/dL	0 (0)	2 (4)	.15
Potassium <3.6 mmol/L	24 (43)	30 (56)	.18
hCG, median (mIU/mL)	131,642	128,992	.27

TSH <0.4 μIU/mL; total bilirubin >1.3 mg/dL; AST >40 U/L or ALT >40 U/L; amylase >108 U/L; lipase >59 U/L. Unless otherwise indicated, all data are presented as n (%). TSH = thyroid-stimulating hormone; AST = aspartate aminotransferase; ALT = alanine aminotransferase; hCG = human chorionic gonadotropin.

Table 3. Course of Hyperemesis Gravidarum Before and After Randomization According to Study Drug

Randomization	Corticosteroids (n = 56)	Placebo (n = 54)	P value
Before randomization			
Number of ER visits	1.3 ± 0.7	1.6 ± 1.0	.07
Duration of hyperemesis (d)	20 ± 21.7	19.5 ± 23.6	.90
After randomization			
Number of ER visits	0.7 ± 1.2	0.5 ± 1.0	.44
Number of admissions	1.9 ± 1.8	1.6 ± 1.0	.32
Women rehospitalized, n (%)	19 (34%)	19 (35%)	.89
Hospital days, first admission	1.9 ± 0.9	2.2 ± 1.2	.47
Total hospital days, all admissions	7.6 ± 18.0	4.3 ± 4.3	.18

Unless otherwise indicated, all data are presented as mean ± SD. ER = emergency room.

who required readmission, 11 in the placebo group and 8 in the corticosteroid group were rehospitalized within 2 weeks of their first admission (P = .33).

Shown in Table 4 are pregnancy complications in women randomized to corticosteroids compared with placebo. There were no significant differences between the study groups. Similarly, neonatal outcomes were not different (Table 5). There was one stillborn fetus during the trial; this occurred in a woman who received corticosteroids. This patient had 6 admissions for hyperemesis gravidarum, the last at 27 weeks' gestation, and the fetal death occurred at 29 weeks. The infant weighed 1090 g and was delivered with a nuchal umbilical cord and no other findings. One woman in the placebo group delivered an infant with microcephaly. This infant weighed 1144 g and was delivered at 27 weeks due to spontaneous labor.

DISCUSSION

The addition of parenteral and oral corticosteroids to the treatment of pregnant women with hyperemesis gravida-

Table 4. Pregnancy Complications in Relation to Corticosteroids or Placebo Treatment of Hyperemesis Gravidarum

Complication	Corticosteroids (n = 56)	Placebo (n = 54)	P value
Spontaneous abortion	2 (4)	3 (6)	.62
Gestational diabetes	3 (5)	3 (6)	.96
Pregnancy hypertension	4 (7)	8 (15)	.20
Preterm delivery ≤36 wk	7 (13)	4 (7)	.37
Cesarean delivery			
Primary	6 (11)	13 (24)	.06
Repeat	4 (7)	6 (11)	.47

All data are presented as n (%).

1252

Table 5. Neonatal Outcomes in Relation to Maternal Therapy for Hyperemesis Gravidarum

Outcome	Corticosteroids ($n = 56$)	Placebo ($n = 54$)	P value
Infant girl	36 (64)	30 (56)	.35
Major anomaly	0	1 (2)	.31
Birth weight (g)			
Mean ± SD	3124 ± 617	3038 ± 834	.55
<1000 g	0	2 (4)	.15
<1500 g	1 (2)	4 (7)	.16
<2500 g	7 (13)	5 (9)	.56
Fetal growth restriction*	7 (13)	10 (19)	.36
Stillborn fetus	1 (2)	0	.32
Neonatal death	0	0	–

Unless otherwise indicated, all data are presented as n (%).

*Birthweight <10th percentile for gestational age.

rum had no appreciable effect—neither beneficial nor deleterious—on the course of hyperemesis or pregnancy outcome. Specifically, the primary outcome in our study, rehospitalization for hyperemesis, occurred in 34% of women who received corticosteroids compared with 35% in women who received placebo. We are disappointed with this result because we had hoped that corticosteroids would prove useful in the management of a common and very difficult to cure complication of pregnancy. It has been argued, however, that no single therapy can be shown to be beneficial because hyperemesis gravidarum is an obstetrical syndrome with several etiologic factors.[14] This may account for much of the frustration in the treatment of hyperemesis gravidarum. It might also be argued that our sample size was too small because it was based on an overly optimistic improvement in the primary outcome from 30% to 5%. We cannot disagree with this argument; however, we point out that the lack of a trend in the proportion of women rehospitalized in this study makes it unlikely that a larger sample size would have revealed a significant benefit for corticosteroid therapy.

Corticosteroids are a logical choice for treatment of nausea and vomiting due to pregnancy because they have been used effectively as an antiemetic in oncology patients.[11,12] Indeed, this use prompted Nelson-Piercy et al[10] to use corticosteroids in four women with refractory hyperemesis gravidarum. These investigators followed this experience with a randomized, placebo-controlled trial of prednisolone in 24 women and found no significant improvement in the frequency of vomiting.[15]

Safari et al,[13] in the only other randomized trial of corticosteroids for hyperemesis gravidarum, assessed the use of oral methylprednisolone versus promethazine in a total of 40 women and concluded that methylprednisolone was superior. However, there was no significant difference in the number of women in each group who stopped vomiting within 2 days of initiating therapy. Fewer women who received methylprednisolone, however, required readmission within 2 weeks (five women who received promethazine versus none who received methylprednisolone). This is contrary to our findings. The study by Safari et al differs from ours in several ways: their study groups each received one drug oral therapy (methylprednisolone or promethazine), whereas our patients received two medications (metoclopramide and promethazine) in addition to the corticosteroid or placebo regimen. Also, our regimen was administered intravenously until an oral regimen was tolerated. Study drug assignment during subsequent admissions was identical to that used for the initial admission, whereas Safari et al allowed crossover. The two studies were similar in that they were conducted in a randomized, double-blind fashion with a 2-week steroid taper.

In a recent evidence-based review of pharmacologic therapy for hyperemesis gravidarum, Magee et al[16] concluded that the pooled results from the literature failed to show that corticosteroids reduced the number of readmissions for hyperemesis gravidarum. Our results support this conclusion.

REFERENCES

1. Miller F. Nausea and vomiting in pregnancy: The problem of perception—Is it really a disease? Am J Obstet Gynecol 2002;186:S182–3.

2. Bennett TA, Kotelchuck M, Cox CE, Tucker MJ, Nadeau DA. Pregnancy-associated hospitalizations in the United States in 1991 and 1992: A comprehensive view of maternal morbidity. Am J Obstet Gynecol 1998;178:346–54.

3. Mazzotta P, Maltepe C, Navioz Y, Magee LA, Koren G. Attitudes, management and consequences of nausea and vomiting of pregnancy in the United States and Canada. Int J Gynecol Obstet 2000;70:359–65.

4. Lavin PJM, Smith D, Kori SH, Ellenberger C. Wernicke's encephalopathy: A predictable complication of hyperemesis gravidarum. Obstet Gynecol 1983;62:13S–15.

5. Fukada Y, Ohta S, Mizuno K, Hoshi K. Rhabdomyolysis secondary to hyperemesis gravidarum. Acta Obstet Gynecol Scand 1999;78:71–3.

6. Robinson JN, Banerjee R, Thiet MP. Coagulopathy secondary to vitamin K deficiency in hyperemesis gravidarum. Obstet Gynecol 1998;92:673–5.

7. Chin RKH, Lao TT. Low birth weight and hyperemesis gravidarum. Eur J Obstet Gynecol Reprod Biol 1988;28:179–83.

8. Geiger CJ, Fahrenbuch DM, Healy FJ. Bendectin in the treatment of nausea and vomiting of pregnancy. Obstet Gynecol 1959;14:688–90.

1253

9. Koren G, Levichek Z. The teratogenicity of drugs for nausea and vomiting of pregnancy: Perceived versus true risk. Am J Obstet Gynecol 2002;186:S248–52.

10. Nelson-Piercy C, de Swiet M. Corticosteroids for the treatment of hyperemesis gravidarum. Br J Obstet Gynaecol 1994;101:1013–5.

11. Italian Group for Antiemetic Research. Dexamethasone, granisetron, or both for the prevention of nausea and vomiting during chemotherapy for cancer. N Engl J Med 1995;332:1–5.

12. Italian Group for Antiemetic Research. Dexamethasone alone or in combination with ondansetron for the prevention of delayed nausea and vomiting induced by chemotherapy. N Engl J Med 2000;342:1554–9.

13. Safari HR, Fassett MJ, Souter IC, Alsulyman OM, Goodwin TM. The efficacy of methylprednisolone in the treatment of hyperemesis gravidarum: A randomized, double-blind, controlled study. Am J Obstet Gynecol 1998;179: 921–4.

14. Goodwin TM. Nausea and vomiting of pregnancy: An obstetric syndrome. Am J Obstet Gynecol 2002;186: S184–9.

15. Nelson-Piercy C, Fayers P, de Swiet M. Randomised, double-blind, placebo-controlled trial of corticosteroids for the treatment of hyperemesis gravidarum. Br J Obstet Gynaecol 2001;108:9–15.

16. Magee LA, Mazzotta P, Koren G. Evidence-based view of safety and effectiveness of pharmacologic therapy for nausea and vomiting of pregnancy (NVP). Am J Obstet Gynecol 2002;186:S256–61.

Address reprint requests to: Nicole P. Yost, MD, University of Texas Southwestern Medical Center, Department of Obstetrics and Gynecology, 5323 Harry Hines Boulevard, Dallas, TX 75390-9032; E-mail: nicole.yost@utsouthwestern.edu.

Received June 10, 2003. Received in revised form August 11, 2003. Accepted August 14, 2003.

Observational study: template

The following template, based on the STROBE statement (www.strobe-statement.org), can be used to critically appraise and evaluate the evidence in published papers reporting an observational study.

A. Title and abstract

1. Is the study design (i.e. cohort, case–control or cross-sectional study) clearly identified in the title?
2. Does the abstract provide a balanced summary of the study design, methods, results and conclusions as well as any major limitations?

B. Introduction

1. Is there a proper description of the scientific background and rationale for the current investigation? Has all the relevant information from any previous studies and other available evidence been included?
2. Is the primary objective of the current investigation indicated, and are secondary objectives described? Were all the objectives pre-specified? If a cohort study, were there any modifications to the original study protocol, including the formulation of additional objectives, following the publication of new evidence after the cohort study was initiated?

C. Methods

1. **Study design** Is the study design described adequately? In particular, is the type of study identified, and a description provided of the study setting and location as well as any relevant dates (including periods of recruitment, exposure, follow-up and data collection)?
2. **Participants**
   a) Are eligibility criteria (inclusion and exclusion) provided for the study participants? Are the sources and methods of selection of participants described?
   b) If a case–control study, is the rationale for the choice of cases and controls explained?
   c) If a cohort study, is the method of follow-up described?
   d) Was the study conducted using an appropriate spectrum of participants?
   e) If the study was matched, is information provided on the matching criteria and the number of exposed and unexposed participants (cohort study) or controls per case (case–control study)?
3. **Variables**
   a) Is there a clear description of outcomes, exposures, predictors, potential confounders and effect modifiers (with details of methods of assessment and diagnostic criteria, if applicable)?
   b) Are details provided on the comparability of assessment methods if there is more than one group?
4. **Bias** Have any efforts been made to address potential sources of bias? Are these fully described?
5. **Sample size** Is there a full explanation of how the study size was determined?
6. **Statistical methods**
   a) Is there a description of how numerical variables were handled in the analysis, including any choice of groupings?
   b) Are all the statistical methods used, including those adopted to control for confounding, fully described?
   c) If relevant, are the methods used to examine subgroups and interactions described?
   d) Is there a description of how missing data have been dealt with in all relevant analyses?
   e) Is there a description of how losses to follow-up (cohort studies), matching (case–control studies) or sampling strategy (cross-sectional studies) have been dealt with?
   f) Are all sensitivity analyses fully described?

D. Results

1. **Participant numbers and dates**
   a) Is there a report of the number of individuals included at each stage of the study (e.g. the numbers who are potentially eligible, are examined for eligibility, are confirmed eligible, are included in the study, completed follow-up and are included in the analysis), preferably through the use of a flow chart?
   b) If relevant, are reasons for nonparticipation at any stage documented?

Medical Statistics at a Glance Workbook, First Edition. Aviva Petrie and Caroline Sabin.

2. **Descriptive data**
   a) Are the characteristics of study participants (demographic, clinical and social) and information on exposures and potential confounders provided?
   b) Is there an indication of the number of participants with missing data for each variable of interest?
   c) If a cohort study, is the follow-up time summarised (e.g. average and total amount)?
3. **Main results**
   a) *Main outcome measures.* Is there full information on outcomes, for example the number of outcome events or summary measures over time (cohort studies), numbers in each exposure category or summary measures of exposure (case–control studies) or number of outcome events or summary measures (cross-sectional studies)?
   b) *Magnitude of effects of interest.* Are unadjusted estimates and, if applicable, confounder-adjusted estimates provided?
   c) *Precision of effects of interest.* Is there an indication of the precision (e.g. 95% confidence intervals) of the estimates?
   d) *If applicable,* is there a clear indication of which confounders were adjusted for in the analysis and why they were selected?
4. **Other analyses** Are the results reported of all other analyses performed, including analyses of subgroups and interactions and any sensitivity analyses?

E. Discussion

1. **Summary of key results**
   a) Is there a summary of the key findings with reference to the study objectives?
   b) Do the results make **biological sense**?
   c) Consider the **confidence interval** for any effect of interest:
      (i) Would you regard the observed effect clinically important (irrespective of whether or not the result of the relevant hypothesis test is statistically significant) if the lower limit of the confidence interval represented the true value of the effect?
      (ii) Would you regard the observed effect clinically important if the upper limit of the confidence interval represented the true value of the effect?
      (iii) Are your answers to the above two points sufficiently similar to declare the results of the study unambiguous and important?
   d) If feasible, have any estimates of relative 'risk' (e.g. odds ratio or relative risk) been translated into absolute 'risks' for a meaningful time period?
2. **Limitations** Is there a discussion of all the study limitations, including the sources of imprecision and the sources and effect (i.e. direction and magnitude) of any potential bias?
3. **Generalisability** Is there a discussion of the generalisability (external validity) of the study findings (i.e. the extent to which the participants are representative of the wider population)?
4. **Interpretation** Are the study findings interpreted in a cautious way, taking full consideration of the study objectives, the limitations of the study, any multiple testing, the results from other similar studies and any other relevant evidence?

F. Other information

1. **Funding** Are the sources of funding documented both for the original study on which the article is based (if relevant) and for the present study, and is the role of the funders described?
2. **Conflict of interest** Is there a clear and transparent conflict-of-interest statement for each of the investigators?

Observational study: Paper 2

The following paper is from *Annals of Surgery* 2011; 254(2): 375–82. Reproduced with permission of Wolters Kluwer Health.

Risk Factors for Mortality in Major Digestive Surgery in the Elderly

A Multicenter Prospective Study

Jean-Jacques Duron, MD,*† Emmanuelle Duron, MD,‡§ Thimothée Dugue, MD,¶ José Pujol, MD,**
Fabrice Muscari, MD,†††‡‡ Denis Collet, MD,§§¶¶ Patrick Pessaux, MD,***††† and
Jean-Marie Hay, MD‡‡‡§§§

Objective: To identify the mortality risk factors of elderly patients (≥65 years old) during major digestive surgery, as defined according to the complexity of the operation.

Background: In the aging populations of developed countries, the incidence rate of major digestive surgery is currently on the rise and is associated with a high mortality rate. Consequently, validated indicators must be developed to improve elderly patients' surgical care and outcomes.

Methods: We acquired data from a multicenter prospective cohort that included 3322 consecutive patients undergoing major digestive surgery across 47 different facilities. We assessed 27 pre-, intra-, and postoperative demographic and clinical variables. A multivariate analysis was used to identify the independent risk factors of mortality in elderly patients (n = 1796). Young patients were used as a control group, and the end-point was defined as 30-day postoperative mortality.

Results: In the entire cohort, postoperative mortality increased significantly among patients aged 65–74 years, and an age ≥65 years was by itself an independent risk factor for mortality (odds ratio [OR], 2.21; 95% confidence interval [CI], 1.36–3.59; $P = 0.001$). The mortality rate among elderly patients was 10.6%. Six independent risk factors of mortality were characteristic of the elderly patients: age ≥85 years (OR, 2.62; 95% CI, 1.08–6.31; $P = 0.032$), emergency (OR, 3.42; 95% CI, 1.67–6.99; $P = 0.001$), anemia (OR, 1.80; 95% CI, 1.02–3.17; $P = 0.041$), white cell count > 10,000/mm^3 (OR, 1.90; 95% CI, 1.08–3.35; $P = 0.024$), ASA class IV (OR, 9.86; 95% CI, 1.77–54.7; $P = 0.009$) and a palliative cancer operation (OR, 4.03; 95% CI, 1.99–8.19; $P < 0.001$).

Conclusion: Characterization of independent validated risk indicators for mortality in elderly patients undergoing major digestive surgery is essential and may lead to an efficient specific workup, which constitutes a necessary step to developing a dedicated score for elderly patients.

(*Ann Surg* 2011;254:375–382)

In developed countries, life expectancy and the elderly population have increased steadily in recent decades.[1–3] In 2008, 32% of the French population was ≥65 years, and 17% was ≥ 75 years of age.[4] Today, major surgical operations are offered to increasing numbers of elderly patients.[5] As in other surgical specialties,[6] the frequency of digestive operations performed in elderly patients,[6] and even in subgroups of older patients (ie, ≥80 or ≥85 years)[7,8] has increased.[7–10] Despite constant advances, these patients' postoperative mortality and morbidity rates remain high,[11] and the preoperative choices for workup often require validated outcome indicators. In this setting, many studies focus exclusively on a particular disease (eg, colon, gastric, or esophageal cancer[12,13]), on a specific operation (eg, colectomy, gastrectomy, esophagectomy, hepatectomy, or pancreatectomy)[14–18] or on an arbitrarily defined age group (eg, octogenarians or nonagenarians).[19–29] Furthermore, data in the literature often differ according to hospital type,[8,30–33] cohort profile (eg, single-center prospective cohort[8,30,33] or mainly male cohort[34]), the definition of the surgery,[31,34] and the definition of the postoperative length of follow-up (postoperative surgical stay,[3,31] 30 days[8,34–36] or longer[37,38]).

In contrast, the study is based on a prospective multicenter cohort of 3322 consecutive patients undergoing major digestive surgery. Using multivariate analysis, the report highlights specific postoperative independent mortality risk factors among patients over 65-year-old, with young patients used as a control group.

PATIENTS AND METHODS

We prospectively enrolled 3322 consecutive patients (1729 males; 52%), mean age 63.8 years (SD 15.3, range 16–99 years), who underwent major digestive surgery. In this cohort, 1796 (54%) patients were over 65 years of age, mean age 75 years (SD 6.7).

Patients underwent surgery between January 01, 2002 and December 31, 2004 in 47 French surgical centers (17 universities [53% of the patients], 27 general [37% of the patients], and 3 private hospitals [10% of the patients]). The average number of patients enrolled by center was 75 ± 63 (median 49, range 0–362). A minimum enrollment of 30 patients per year was necessary for a facility to participate in our study. The centers initiated the enrollment on different dates and participated in the study for different lengths of time.

The end point was mortality during the 30 days after the operation.

The eligibility criteria included patients over the age of 16 who underwent a major digestive operation (defined as "major or major plus" according to Copeland[39] or "complex grade 3, 4, and

*Digestive Surgery and Liver Transplantation Unit, University Hospital Pitie-Salpêtrière, 46-83, Boulevard de l'Hôpital, Paris, France; †Hôpitaux de Paris. Pierre and Marie Curie University, Paris, France; ‡Geriatric Unit, University Hospital Broca, Paris, France; §Hôpitaux de Paris, Descartes University, Paris, France; ¶General and Digestive Surgery Unit, Saint Philibert Hospital, Lomme, France; **General Surgery Unit, Samuel Pozzi Hospital, 9 Boulevard Albert Calmette, Bergerac, France; ††Digestive Surgery Unit, University Hospital Rangueil, Toulouse, France; ‡‡Paul Sabatier University Toulouse, France; §§General and Digestive Surgery Unit, University Hospital Haut-Levesques, Pessac, France; ¶¶Victor Segalene University Bordeaux, France; ***Visceral Surgery Unit, University Hospital Angers, Angers; †††Angers University, France; ‡‡‡General and Digestive Surgery Unit, University Hospital Louis Mourier, Colombes Cedex, France; §§§Hôpitaux de Paris, Paris. Diderot University Paris, Paris, France.

Supported by 3 grants: Haute Autorité de Santé (HAS) GJ/SF/109-05 PR 01-010; Programme Hospitalier de Recherche Clinique (PHRC) Appel d'offre Régional (AOR) 03-01, and Ligue Nationale Contre le Cancer (LNCC) PRC-2003-LNCC/JMH1.
Reprints: Jean Jacques Duron. Service de Chirurgie Digestive et de Transplantation Hépatique. Hôpital de la Pitie Salpetriere, 83 Boulevard de l'Hôpital, 75013 Paris, France. E-mail: jjduron@orange.fr.
ISSN: 0003-4932/11/25402-0375
DOI: 10.1097/SLA.0b013e318226a959

375

5" according to Aust et al[40]) as well as certain other operations (intraperitoneal hyperthermic chemotherapy, bariatric surgery bypass, and strictureplasty). Noneligibility criteria were used to eliminate any living patients without a follow-up within 30 days postoperation (n = 308). Those patients for whom missing data/patients accounted for >3 of all records were excluded (n = 251) from the initial 3881 patient cohort.

RISK FACTORS

With reference to the studies by Copeland, Arozullah and Leung et al,[3,41,42] 27 demographic and clinical variables accounting for their known influence on the perioperative period were recorded: age (± 65 years); gender; emergency (time from admission to operation <24 hours for a nonscheduled operation)[43]; body mass index (BMI) ±30; weight loss (weight loss of >10% body weight in the previous 6 months)[44]; kidney failure (Cockroft <60 mL/minute)[45]; anemia upon admission (hemoglobin <13 g/dL in men and <12 g/dL in women)[46,47]; white cell count upon admission >10,000/mm^3;[43] diabetes (Type I or II); history of heart disease (hypertension, recent myocardial infarction, cardiomyopathy, congestive heart failure, and heart rhythm troubles)[42]; cirrhosis with clinical or histological evidence; history of neurological disease (stroke with or without residual sequelae, Parkinson's disease, dementia); history of pulmonary disease (chronic pulmonary troubles, chronic obstructive pulmonary disease [COPD]) requiring permanent bronchodilator therapy or hospitalizations for treatment[42]; infectious condition upon admission necessitating immediate antibiotic therapy; positive preoperative blood-culture[8]; potential impaired healing due to steroid therapy, cancer chemotherapy or radiotherapy in the previous 6 months[48]; dependence defined by the assistance of another person for some activities coupled with the use of assistive equipment for everyday activities[42]; American Association of Anesthesiologists (ASA) classification encompassing a unique class IV (merging class IV and V)[49]; cancer[35,36]; in the case of cancer, palliative surgery defined as an incomplete intraoperative excision, visceral metastasis or carcinomatosis; type of surgery (open or laparoscopic surgery [including assisted or converted laparoscopic procedures]); blood transfusion ≥4 units during the perioperative period[42]; surgical sites (colorectal, liver–biliary track, esophagus-stomach-intestine, pancreas [categorized according to surgical and anatomical criteria]); length of operation ≥5 hours[50]; parietal surgical postoperative complications (abscess, hematoma, and incisional hernia); deep surgical postoperative complications (abscess, peritonitis, hemorrhage, and anastomotic leakage); minor medical postoperative complications (without any intensive care admission); and severe medical postoperative complications (more than 1 day in the intensive care unit in the absence of any surgical complications).[37,51]

STATISTICAL ANALYSIS

The statistical analysis encompassed several steps using logistic model regressions.

The first step in the entire cohort was a study of the age-based mortality, the continuous age variable being categorized from 35 years in age groups of 10 years, similar to the segmentation used by the World Health Organization (WHO) in patients over the age of 65.[52]

The second step was a prevalence and univariate analysis of the risk factors in ≥65 and <65 years of age.

The third step consisted of a multivariate logistic analysis of mortality that incorporated all risk factors (including age ≥65 years/<65 years) with $P \leq 0.10$ in the univariate analysis (forward stepwise elimination). This multivariate logistic model was then independently applied to the 2 age groups (namely, ≥65 years and <65 years) with the specific risk factors (including age).

The relative risks were expressed as odds ratios (OR) with a 95 (%) confidence interval (CI). In all analyses, $P \leq 0.05$ was considered significant. The missing values were treated according to an imputation procedure, and a postestimation of the model goodness of fit was performed using the C Index and Hosmer-Lemeshow tests. A bootstrapping procedure with 200 replications was used to assess the stability of the model.

Statistical analyses were performed with STATA MP 10.1 software (StataCorp, College Station, TX, USA).

RESULTS

Postoperative mortality. The mortality rate of the global postoperative cohort was 7% (233 of 3322), with a mortality rate of 24% after emergency surgery (114 of 466) versus 4% (119 of 2856) for elective surgery ($P \leq 0.001$). The mortality rates exponentially increased with age across the entire cohort (Fig. 1). The relationship between age and mortality was as follows: postoperative mortality = $0.002 \times \exp (0.63 \times \text{age})$. The mortality increase seemed to be statistically significant in the 65 to 74 years age group ($P \leq 0.03$), and being older than 65 was on its own a significant independent risk factor of mortality (OR, 2.21; 95%CI, 1.36–3.59; $P = 0.001$). In our text, elderly and the elderly group will refer to patients ≥65 year of age, whereas young and the young group will refer to patients <65 years of age. Age was not a significant risk of mortality in the young group, but in the elderly group, belonging to the ≥85-year-old group (mortality 18%) emerged as an independent risk of mortality (OR, 2.62; 95%CI, 1.08–6.31; $P = 0.032$).

The postoperative mortality of elderly patients was 10.6% (191 of 1796) versus 2.7% (42 of 1526) in young patients ($P \leq 0.001$). The mortality after emergency procedures in elderly patients was 33.5% (102 of 304) versus 7.4% (12 of 162) in young patients ($P \leq 0.001$), and the mortality after elective surgery in elderly patients was 6% (89 of 1492) versus 2.2% (30 of 1364) in young patients ($P \leq 0.001$).

The prevalence of demographic and clinical risk factors for mortality among elderly versus young patients, as well as mortality (Tables 1 and 2), were collected from the cohort.

Seventeen risk factors were significantly more common in elderly patients: emergency; anemia; diabetes; kidney failure; history of heart disease; pulmonary disease; neurological disease; potential impaired healing; dependence; ASA class II, III and IV; cancer; palliative cancer surgery; colorectal surgical site [with a remarkably high emergency prevalence of 88% (268 of 304)]; and minor and severe medical complications.

Six risk factors were significantly more common in young patients: BMI < 30;

ASA I; laparoscopic procedures; length of surgery ≥5 hours; and liver–biliary track and pancreatic surgical sites.

Eight risk factors were not significantly different in elderly patients as compared with young patients: gender; weight loss; white cell count >10,000/mm^3; cirrhosis; transfusion; esophagus–stomach–intestine surgical site; and parietal and deep surgical complications.

Our univariate analysis of the risk factors for postoperative death is reported in Table 3.

Four factors that affected the risk of mortality were statistically significant in elderly patients: ASA II, cancer, and colorectal and esophagus–stomach–intestine surgical sites.

Four factors were statistically significant in the young patients: gender, cirrhosis, potential impaired healing, and pancreatic surgical site.

Eighteen factors were statistically significant in both the elderly and young patients: emergency, weight loss, anemia, white cells > 10,000/mm^3; kidney failure; history of cardiac, pulmonary and neurological disease; dependence; infectious disease; ASA III and

376

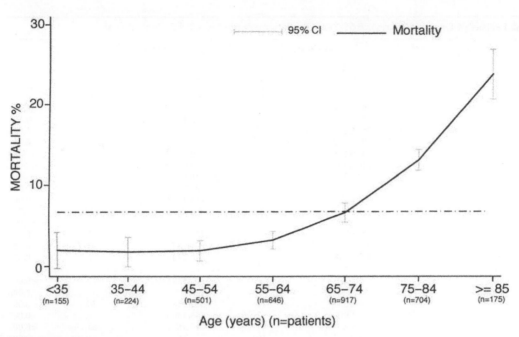

FIGURE 1. Mortality according to age.

IV; open procedure; palliative cancer surgery; transfusion; deep surgical complications; and minor and severe medical complications.

Four risk factors for mortality were not significant in the elderly patients or in the young patients: BMI ≥30; diabetes; length of operation ≥5 hours; and parietal surgical complications.

Overall, our multivariate analysis highlighted 13 independent mortality risk factors (Table 4), as follows. Six factors were characteristic of the elderly patients: age ≥ 85 years; emergency; anemia; white cell count >10,000/mm³; palliative cancer; and ASA IV. Three factors were common to the elderly and young patients: deep surgical complications; minor and severe medical complications. Four other factors were characteristic of the young patients: kidney failure; cirrhosis; dependence; and pancreatic surgical site.

DISCUSSION

First, our study identified a significant increase in study-wide mortality in the 6574 age group across the entire cohort of patients undergoing major digestive surgery, and age ≥65 years was an independent mortality risk factor. Thus, in this type of surgery, the 65-year-old cut-off, consistent with the empirical WHO cut-off for "aged" people[52] that has been used in other studies,[53–56] is objectively relevant for defining elderly patients even though other authors have subjectively chosen to adopt other cut-offs.[19–21,23,24–29,54–56] A comparison of our postoperative mortality rates (7% overall, and 10.6% in elderly patients) with those of other studies is difficult due to the different case profiles (mortality ranging from 1.5%[57] to 14%[22]) and to the often underreported mortality rates of the elderly.[11]

Subsequently, our analysis individualized independent mortality risk factors of elderly and young patients. The prevalence of these factors (except for that of the pancreas site, which is lower) and mortality rates were always either significantly higher or not different in the elderly compared with the young patients (Tables 1 and 2).

In our elderly patients, we individualized 6 characteristic independent mortality risk factors. First, age ≥85 years is clearly a risk factor of death. This age (or other close age cut-offs) was already reported as a risk factor of death,[8,31,58,59] even though some retrospective studies with selection and inclusion biases stress the fact that extreme age on its own is not a risk factor of death.[19–24,27–29,60–62]

Second, ASA class IV, an accepted surgical mortality indicator in the general population,[34,63,64] was revealed as a risk factor of death in our elderly patients. Its higher prevalence in the elderly (6% with a 56% related mortality [Tables 1 and 2]) is due to the frequency of comorbidities[65] resulting from the progressive degradation of all physiological functions[1–3] occurring at the time of operation.[26,27,33,34,65,66] In our elderly group, we retrieved 6% patients ASA IV (Table 1) with 56% related mortality (Table 4). These figures are consistent with reports in the literature that describe high ASA scores as risk factors for mortality in elderly people who have undergone general and digestive surgery.[3,8,26,33,34,63,65]

Third, emergency has high prevalence (17%) and mortality rates (34%; Tables 1 and 2) consistent with reports in the literature[21,27]; this finding may be related to the increased incidence of certain diseases with age (eg, colon and rectal cancers)[7] and to delayed surgical presentation of elderly patients.[2] This elevated mortality rate, as demonstrated by the absence of a significant difference between surgical sites, was not linked to the type of surgery.[66]

Fourth, anemia also showed high prevalence (21%), in line with published figures ranging from 5.5% to 48%,[53,54,67] and a related high mortality (19%)[63] (Tables 1 and 2). Even if the causes of anemia in elderly individuals are multiple,[46,47,67] Knight et al[56] noted that 40% of patients with initial stage and 80% with advanced stage colon cancer suffer from anemia that is associated with a decreased survival rate. Moreover, even moderate anemia might be associated with higher short-term postoperative mortality.[68]

Fifth, in line with our findings, white cell counts were already reported to be linked with postoperative complications in colon cancer surgery[69] and individualized as a risk factor of death in several studies.[40,43]

Sixth, palliative cancer surgery is an independent risk factor for mortality among our elderly patients compared with cancer alone. Cancer prevalence (14%) is associated with a high mortality rate (21%) with no significant difference related to operative site. In the

377

TABLE 1. Risk Factors of Death (30 days). <65-Year-Old Patients/≥65-Year-Old Patients Prevalence

Risk Factors	<65 Years N (1526) Yes/No	% (46)	≥65 Years N (1796) Yes/No	% (54)	P	N
Gender female	708/818	46	885/911	49	0.112	3322
Emergency	162/1364	11	304/1492	17	**<0.001**	3322
Weight loss>10 kg	171/1351	11	175/1616	10	0.172	3313
BMI ≥ 30	260/1230	17	234/1487	14	**0.003**	3211
Anemia	173/1347	11	381/1414	21	**<0.001**	3315
White cell count >10,000/mm^3	334/1191	22	439/1355	24	0.84	3319
Diabetes	116/1398	8	255/11515	14	**<0.001**	3284
Kidney failure	131/1261	9	799/709	53	**<0.001**	2900
Heart disease	313/1205	21	1064/717	60	**<0.001**	3299
Pulmonary disease	59/1424	4	138/1583	8	**<0.001**	3204
Cirrhosis	34/1484	2	44/1741	2	0.731	3303
Neurologic disease	72/1436	5	172/1594	10	**<0.001**	3274
Dependence	49/1453	3	217/1544	12	**<0.001**	3263
Potential impaired healing	307/1206	10	295/1474	17	**<0.001**	3282
Infectious condition	232/1198	16	330/1348	20	**0.013**	3108
ASA						
ASA I	561/841	40	190/1493	11	**<0.001**	751
ASA II	671/731	48	887/796	53	**<0.008**	1558
ASA III	149/1253	11	503/1180	30	**<0.001**	652
ASA IV	21/1381	2	103/1580	6	**<0.001**	124
Cancer	719/807	47	1171/624	65	**<0.001**	3319
Palliative cancer operation	146/1373	10	247/1540	14	**<0.001**	3306
Laparoscopy	469/1048	31	309/1473	17	**<0.001**	3299
Transfusion	71/1437	5	89/1679	5	0.685	3276
Surgical site						
Colon rectum	863/663	57	1197/599	67	**<0.001**	2060
Liver–biliary tract	251/1275	16	206/1590	11	**<0.001**	457
Oesophagus–stomach–intestin	213/1313	14	230/1566	13	0.356	443
Pancreas	199/1327	13	163/1633	9	**0.003**	362
Operation length ≥5 hours	302/1209	20	286/1484	16	**0.004**	3281
Parietal surgical complications	117/1399	8	159/1613	9	0.207	3288
Deep surgical complications	191/1328	13	203/1568	11	0.333	3290
Minor medical complications	107/1334	7	240/1464	14	**<0.001**	3145
Severe medical complications	86/1356	6	163/1547	10	**<0.001**	3152
Mortality						
Median of patients/variable: 3286	42/1484	2.7	191/1605	10.6	**<0.001**	3322
Missing patients/variable: mean: 75, median: 23, range: 0–422						

Bold and italic values indicate that $P \leq 0.05$ was considered significant.

TABLE 2. Significant Risk Factors Postoperative Mortality Prevalence. <65-Year-Old/>65-Year-Old Patients

Risk Factors	Deaths: <65-year-old Patients N	%	Death: >65-year-old Patients N	%	P
Emergency	12/162	7	102/304	34	**<0.001**
Kidney failure	11/131	9	108/799	14	<0.120
Cirrhosis	7/34	21	8/44	18	1
Anemia	18/173	10	73/381	19	**<0.009**
White cell count>10,000/mm^3	20/314	6	106/333	24	**<0.001**
Dependence	14/49	29	60/217	27	<0.860
ASA IV	10/21	48	58/103	56	**<0.480**
Palliative cancer operation	12/143	8	51/247	21	**<0.010**
Surgical site pancreas	12/199	6	13/163	7	0.061
Deep surgical complications	20/191	10	55/203	27	<0.001
Minor medical complications	9/107	8	68/240	28	**<0.001**
Severe medical complications	8/86	9	42/143	26	**<0.002**

Only statistically significant risk factors from the multivariate analysis are reported in this table. Bold values indicate that $P \leq 0.05$ was considered significant.

378

TABLE 3. Risk Factors of Death (30 days). <65-Year-Old Patients/≥65-Years-Old Patients Univariate Analysis

Risk Factors	<65 Years				≥65 Years			
	Death Yes/No	OR	95%CI	P	Death Yes/No	OR	95%CI	P
Gender female	13/695	0.50	0.26–0.98	**0.046**	87/798	0.84	0.62–1.14	0.276
Emergency	12/150	3.68	1.83–7.42	**<0.001**	102/202	7.96	5.77–10.0	**<0.001**
weight loss	12/157	4.37	2.34–7.18	**<0.001**	28/147	1.82	11.17–3.60	**<0.001**
BMI ≥ 30	7/253	1.00	0.43–2.29	0.993	25/209	1.16	0.73–1.81	0.518
Anemia	18/155	6.68	3.52–12.66	**<0.001**	73/308	2.60	1.89–3.57	**<0.001**
White cell count >10,000/mm^3	20/314	3.38	1.82–6.28	**<0.001**	106/333	4.75	3.48–6.48	**<0.001**
Diabetes	4/112	1.25	0.52–3.48	0.646	21/234	0.73	0.45–1.18	0.213
Kidney failure	11/120	4.35	2.09–9.03	**<0.001**	108/691	2.48	1.71–3.60	**<0.001**
Heart disease	15/298	2.19	1.15–4.18	**<0.001**	131/933	1.65	1.19–2.30	**0.003**
Pulmonary disease	7/52	5.34	2.26–12.59	**<0.001**	28/110	2.41	1.54–3.77	**<0.001**
Cirrhosis	7/27	10.73	4.37–26.30	**<0.001**	8/36	1.90	0.87–4.15	*0.106*
Neurologic disease	8/64	5.15	2.29–11.58	**<0.001**	41/131	3.12	2.11–4.61	**<0.001**
Dependence	14/35	20.35	9.87–41.98	**<0.001**	60/157	4.33	3.05–6.15	**<0.001**
Potential impaired healing	20/287	3.45	9.87–41.98	**<0.001**	39/256	1.35	0.92–1.97	0.115
Infectious condition	12/220	2.36	1.18–4.74	**0.022**	59/271	2.33	1.66–3.28	**<0.001**
ASA								
ASA I	4/557				2/188			
ASA II	14/657	2.96	0.05–0.91	*0.056*	47/840	5.25	11.3–21.84	**0.022**
ASA III	10/139	10.01	33.1–32.41	**<0.001**	70/433	15.19	3.68–62.61	**<0.001**
ASA IV	10/11	126.59	34.3–46.6	**<0.001**	58/45	121.15	28.5–514.1	**<0.001**
Cancer	26/691	1.86	0.99–3.49	*0.054*	105/1066	0.61	0.45–0.83	**0.002**
Palliative cancer operation	12/134	4.00	2.00–8.01	**<0.001**	51/196	2.64	1.85–3.76	**<0.001**
Laparoscopy	6/463	0.36	0.15–0.87	**0.023**	12/297	0.29	0.16–0.53	**<0.001**
Transfusion	3/16	6.97	1.95–24.90	**0.007**	7/19	3.21	1.33–7.75	**0.009**
Surgical site								
Liver–biliary track	5/246				7/199			
Colon–rectum	15/848	0.87	0.31–2.41	*0.790*	131/1066	3.49	1.60–7.58	**0.002**
Oesophagus–stomach–intestin	10/203	2.42	0.81–7.20	0.111	40/190	5.98	2.61–13.68	**<0.001**
Pancreas	12/187	3.15	1.09–9.11	**0.034**	13/150	2.46	0.95–6.32	0.061
Operation length ≥ 5h	9/293	1.09	0.51–2.31	0.81	26/260	0.81	0.52–1.25	0.34
Parietal surgical complications	5/112	1.79	1.40–6.33	0.233	23/136	1.64	1.02–2.64	0.038
Deep surgical complications	20/171	6.5	0.68–4.67	**<0.001**	55/148	4.48	3.12–6.43	**<0.001**
Minor medical complications	9/98	4.28	1.96–9.33	**<0.001**	68/172	5.22	3.70–7.37	**<0.001**
Severe medical complications	8/78	4.68	2.14–11.02	**0.001**	42/121	3.69	2.48–5.46	**<0.001**

OR indicates odd ratio; 95%CI: 95% confidence interval. Bold and italic values indicate that $P \leq 0.05$ was considered significant.

literature dealing specifically with major digestive surgery in the elderly, cancer is rarely reported as a risk factor for death.[70] Abbas et al[27] reported the absence of any difference in long-term survival rates for octogenarians from cancer-versus non–cancer-associated major digestive surgery. Khuri and Reiss reported that "disseminated cancer or inoperable cancer" (close to our definition) may be short- and long-term risk factors for mortality.[37,59]

In our cohort, deep surgical complications and minor as well as severe postoperative medical complications were common risk factors for mortality among elderly and young patients.

The prevalence of deep surgical complications was not statistically different in elderly and young patients, in contrast to mortality, which was higher in elderly patients (27%; Tables 1 and 2). These results may be explained by the similarity of the surgical procedures in young and elderly people, resulting in an equal number of deep surgical complications leading to more severe consequences in elderly people. In line with the literature,[8,13,34,58] our prevalence of postoperative minor (14%) and severe medical complications (10%) was high in elderly patients. The associated mortality rates were 28% and 26%, respectively. Several studies with different baseline characteristics and inclusion criteria resulting in relatively low mortality rates emphasized postoperative complications as major risk factors of mortality[34,37,58] and pointed to some of them as main opportunities for improving care for elderly people.[56] Nevertheless, in our high mortality elderly group, the workup of preoperative predictors of mortality remains an essential target.[3,62,65]

In young patients, 4 characteristic independent factors of postoperative mortality were identified: kidney failure, cirrhosis, dependence, and pancreatic surgical site.

These risk factors, compared with other series,[8] did not appear in our elderly patients despite similar or even greater prevalence than in young patients. The absence of kidney failure and cirrhosis as risk factors in our group of elderly patients may be related to the lack of a severity scale to interpret our binary data. Dependence, evaluated according to attainable criteria in surgical settings, probably does not correspond to an identical status in the elderly and young patients.[1,71–73] The risk linked to the pancreatic surgical site results from the higher frequencies of these high-risk major operations in young patients.[74]

The 6 specific elderly patient predictors of death cannot be equally affected in the preoperative period. Two predictors, age ≥85 years and ASA class IV, are clearly not open to modifications. The 4 other predictors, either directly (preoperative treatments for anemia and white cell count) or indirectly (preventive measures for emergency and palliative cancer surgery), could benefit from an efficient specific workup.

Regarding anemia, preoperative transfusions must, except for emergency situations, generally be reserved for cases of severe

379

TABLE 4. Risk Factors of Death. 65<Year-Old Patients>65-Year-Old Patients Multivariate Analysis

Risk Factors	<65 ANS			>65 ANS		
	OR	CI95%	P	OR	CI95%	P
Age > 85				2.62	1.08–6.31	**0.032**
Emergency				3.42	1.67–6.99	**0.001**
Kidney failure	11.44	2.25–57.96	**0.003**			
Cirrrhosis	13.25	2.11–82.89	**0.006**			
Anemia				1.80	1.02–3.17	**0.041**
White cell count >10,000/mm^3				1.90	1.08–3.35	**0.024**
Dependence	5.17	1.09–28.09	**0.047**			
ASA IV				9.86	1.77–54.7	**0.009**
Palliative cancer operation				4.03	1.99–8.19	**<0.001**
Surgical site: pancreas	7.78	1.59–37.95	**0.011**			
Deep surgical complications	63.13	5.51–723.33	**0.001**	51.59	18.02–147.68	**<0.001**
Minor medical complications	40.04	2.78–575.49	**0.007**	40.58	15.08–109.19	**<0.001**
Severe medical complications	108.08	8.59–13558.8	**<0.001**	23.36	8.21–66.46	**<0.001**

OR indicates odd ratio; 95%CI, 95% confidence interval; <65 years: C index 0.98 Hosmer–Lemeshow, $P = 0.999$; >65 years: C index 0.93 Hosmer–Lemeshow, $P = 0.728$. Bold values indicate that $P \leq 0.05$ was considered significant.

anemia.[75,76] Nevertheless, the preoperative hematocrit might influence the 30-day postoperative mortality in elderly patients requiring intraoperative transfusion during major noncardiac surgery.[77] Before elective surgery, recombinant hematopoetin may be an option, as several studies show its efficacy.[53–56]

A white cell count >10,000/mm^3, as a risk factor of death, reinforces the conclusion of the study by Silber et al[78] that showed that elderly digestive surgery requires preoperative antibiotics.

As recommended almost 2 decades ago,[79] the high emergency mortality rate of elderly patients can only be decreased by an earlier diagnostic strategy (eg, anemia assessment[70,80]) leading to more frequent elective operations,[2,3] particularly in elderly patients undergoing colorectal surgery whose inequity in treatment is recognized.[81]

In the same way, concerning cancer, 2 courses of action can be proposed. First, the severity of palliative resections in elderly patients, frequently referred with advanced stages of cancer,[2,13] could benefit from less-invasive approaches. Thus, in place of surgery, palliative stent placements may be an efficient definitive option.[82,83] Second, in the long run, systematic screening campaigns, which are efficient in cases of colorectal cancer in patients under 75,[84] could promote the early discovery of initial-stage tumors with more favorable prognoses. Such an approach is supported by the similar survival rates after oncological curative surgery in old and young patients.[9]

In our study, several limitations have to be emphasized: (1) potentially important markers were probably insufficiently assessed (eg, as nutritional status indicators,[65] frailty or prefrailty markers[38,85]); (2) even if our cohort is prospective and multicenter-based, selection biases are possible, because on the one hand, enrolled patients and their families agreed to the proposed major operation, and on the other hand, a relative surgical abstention from high-risk operations (eg, pancreas and liver)[62] is possible; and (3) as in similar studies,[8,34] our multivariate analysis only highlights isolated independent death indicators. It does not evaluate, as does a score,[86,87] the association of several factors open or not open to improvements.

Thus, a comprehensive geriatric-specific and oncological preoperative assessment is essential in elderly patients[2,38,62,65,88] to allow the further individualization of indicators of death, which can lead to an efficient specific risk-based workup. Moreover, these indicators are essential to develop and validate a scoring system according to a precise and dedicated methodology. This score for elderly patients would be useful in predicting the risk of death for individuals and, for populations, in comparing the performance of hospitals, surgical units, and/or surgeons.

ACKNOWLEDGMENTS

We wish to thank the contributing surgeons and participating subjects at Fédération de Recherche En Chirurgie (FRENCH): Brassier, Didier (Aulnay/Bois); Collet, Denis (Pessac/Bordeaux); De Calan, Loic (Tours); Decker, Georges (Luxembourg); Bakoto, C (Chateauroux); Descottes, Bernard (Limoges); Demaizieres, François (Paray-le-Monial); Desrousseaux, Bruno (Lomme); Desvignes, Gerard (Montargis Amilly); Dillin Christian (Thonon les Bains); Ducerf, Christian (Lyon); Dugue, Timothée (Lomme); Evrard, Serge (Bordeaux); Fabre Xavier (Cholet); Flamant, Yves (Colombes); Fingerhut, Abe (Poissy); Fourtanier, Gilles (Toulouse); Gabelle, Philippe (Grenoble); Gaignant, Alain (Limoges); Gayet, Brice (Paris); Hennet, Henri (Romorantin); Herbiere, Patrick (Albi). Herjean, Marion (Valenciennes); Ianelli, Antonio (Menton); Jaeck, Daniel (Strasbourg); Kohlmann, Gerard (Corbeil-Essonne); Laborde, Yves (Pau); Lehur, Paul-Antoine (Nantes); Langlois-Zantain, Odile (Montluçon); Leynaud, Gérard (Montluçon); Merad, Fehti (Eaubonne Alger); Michot Francis (Rouen); Oberlin, Philippe (Villeneuve St Georges); Pellissier Edouard (Besançon); Pessaux, Patrick (Angers); Peyrard, Pierre (Compiegne); Philippe, Olivier (Orange); Pujol José (Bergerac); Regimbeau, Jean-Marc (Amiens); Rey, Claude (Vernon); Sage, Michel (Auxerre); Segol, Philippe (Caen); Tarla, Emmanuel (Cannes); Tison, Marc (Dunkerque); Triboulet, Jean-Pierre (Lille); Troalen, Karen (Gonesse); Vacher, Bernard (Argenteuil); Veyrieres, Michel (Pontoise).

REFERENCES

1. Richardson JD, Cocanour CS, Kern JA, et al. Perioperative risk assessment in elderly and high-risk patients. J Am Coll Surg. 2004;199:133–146.
2. Seymour DG. Gastrointestinal surgery in old age: issues of equality and quality. Gut. 1997;41:427–429.
3. Leung JM, Dzankic S. Relative importance of preoperative health status versus intraoperative factors in predicting postoperative adverse outcomes in geriatric surgical patients. J Am Geriatr Soc. 2001;49:1080–1085.
4. www.insee.fr.strutures par age des populations maculines et feminines.
5. Etzioni DA, Liu JH, Maggard MA, et al. The aging population and its impact on the surgery workforce. Ann Surg. 2003;238:170–177.
6. Colorectal Cancer Collaborative Group. Surgery for colorectal cancer in elderly patients: a systematic review. Lancet. 2000;356(9234):968–974.
7. de Rijke JM, Schouten LJ, Hillen HF, et al. Cancer in the very elderly Dutch population. Cancer. 2000;89:1121–1133.
8. Turrentine FE, Wang H, Simpson VB, et al. Surgical risk factors, morbidity, and mortality in elderly patients. J Am Coll Surg. 2006;203:865–877.

380

9. Monson K, Litvak DA, Bold RJ. Surgery in the aged population: surgical oncology. *Arch Surg*. 2003;138:1061–1067.

10. Pofahl WE, Pories WJ. Current status and future directions of geriatric general surgery. *J Am Geriatr Soc*. 2003;51(7 Suppl):S351-S354.

11. Finlayson EV, Birkmeyer JD. Operative mortality with elective surgery in older adults. *Eff Clin Pract*. 2001;4:172–177.

12. Alexiou C, Beggs D, Salama FD, et al. Surgery for esophageal cancer in elderly patients: the view from Nottingham. *J Thorac Cardiovasc Surg*. 1998;116:545–553.

13. Latkauskas T, Rudinskaite G, Kurtinaitis J, et al. The impact of age on postoperative outcomes of colorectal cancer patients undergoing surgical treatment. *BMC Cancer*. 2005;5:153.

14. Arenal JJ, Benito C, Concejo MP, et al. Colorectal resection and primary anastomosis in patients aged 70 and older: prospective study. *Eur J Surg*. 1999;165:593–597.

15. Poon RT, Law SY, Chu KM, et al. Esophagectomy for carcinoma of the esophagus in the elderly: results of current surgical management. *Ann Surg*. 1998;227:357–364.

16. Wu YL, Yu JX, Xu B. Safe major abdominal operations: hepatectomy, gastrectomy and pancreatoduodenectomy in elder patients. *World J Gastroenterol*. 2004;10:1995–1997.

17. Aldrighetti L, Arru M, Caterini R, et al. Impact of advanced age on the outcome of liver resection. *World J Surg*. 2003;27:1149–1154.

18. Coniglio A, Tiberio GA, Busti M, et al. Surgical treatment for gastric carcinoma in the elderly. *J Surg Oncol*. 2004;88:201–205.

19. Sohn TA, Yeo CJ, Cameron JL, et al. Should pancreaticoduodenectomy be performed in octogenarians? *J Gastrointest Surg*. 1998;2:207–216.

20. Ackermann RJ, Vogel RL, Johnson LA, et al. Surgery in nonagenarians: morbidity, mortality, and functional outcome. *J Fam Pract*. 1995;40:129–135.

21. Bufalari A, Ferri M, Cao P, et al. Surgical care in octogenarians. *Br J Surg*. 1996;83:1783–1787.

22. Walsh TH. Audit of outcome of major surgery in the elderly. *Br J Surg*. 1996;83:92–97.

23. Burns-Cox N, Campbell WB, van Nimmen BA, et al. Surgical care and outcome for patients in their nineties. *Br J Surg*. 1997;84:496–498.

24. Rigberg D, Cole M, Hiyama D, et al. Surgery in the nineties. *Am Surg*. 2000;66:813–816.

25. Zerbib P, Kulick JF, Lebuffe G, et al. Emergency major abdominal surgery in patients over 85 years of age. *World J Surg*. 2005;29:820–825.

26. Tan KY, Chen CM, Ng C, et al. Which octogenarians do poorly after major open abdominal surgery in our Asian population? *World J Surg*. 2006;30:547–552.

27. Abbas S, Booth M. Major abdominal surgery in octogenarians. *N Z Med J*. 2003;116(1172):U402.

28. Warner MA, Hosking MP, Lobdell CM, et al. Surgical procedures among those greater than or equal to 90 years of age. A population-based study in Olmsted County, Minnesota, 1975-1985. *Ann Surg*. 1988; 207:380–386.

29. Spivak H, Maele DV, Friedman I, et al. Colorectal surgery in octogenarians. *J Am Coll Surg*. 1996;183:46–50.

30. Khuri SF, Najjar SF, Daley J, et al. Comparison of surgical outcomes between teaching and nonteaching hospitals in the Department of Veterans Affairs. *Ann Surg*. 2001;234:370–382.

31. Polanczyk CA, Marcantonio E, Goldman L, et al. Impact of age on perioperative complications and length of stay in patients undergoing noncardiac surgery. *Ann Intern Med*. 2001;134:637–643.

32. Tekkis PP, Prytherch DR, Kocher HM, et al. Development of a dedicated risk-adjustment scoring system for colorectal surgery (colorectal POSSUM). *Br J Surg*. 2004;91:1174–1182.

33. McNicol L, Story DA, Leslie K, et al. Postoperative complications and mortality in older patients having non-cardiac surgery at three Melbourne teaching hospitals. *Med J Aust*. 2007;186:447–452.

34. Hamel MB, Henderson WG, Khuri SF, et al. Surgical outcomes for patients aged 80 and older: morbidity and mortality from major noncardiac surgery. *J Am Geriatr Soc*. 2005;53:424–429.

35. Henderson WG, Khuri SF, Mosca C, et al. Comparison of risk-adjusted 30day postoperative mortality and morbidity in Department of Veterans Affairs hospitals and selected university medical centers: general surgical operations in men. *J Am Coll Surg*. 2007;204:1103–1114.

36. Fink AS, Hutter MM, Campbell DC, Jr., et al. Comparison of risk-adjusted 30-day postoperative mortality and morbidity in Department of Veterans Affairs hospitals and selected university medical centers: general surgical operations in women. *J Am Coll Surg*. 2007;204:1127–1136.

37. Khuri SF, Henderson WG, DePalma RG, et al. Determinants of long-term survival after major surgery and the adverse effect of postoperative complications. *Ann Surg*. 2005;242:326–341.

38. McGory ML, Kao KK, Shekelle PG, et al. Developing quality indicators for elderly surgical patients. *Ann Surg*. 2009;250:338–347.

39. Copeland GP, Sagar P, Brennan J, et al. Risk-adjusted analysis of surgeon performance: a 1-year study. *Br J Surg*. 1995;82:408–411.

40. Aust JB, Henderson W, Khuri S, et al. The impact of operative complexity on patient risk factors. *Ann Surg*. 2005;241:1024–1027.

41. Copeland GP, Jones D, Walters M. POSSUM: a scoring system for surgical audit. *Br J Surg*. 1991;78:355–360.

42. Arozullah AM, Daley J, Henderson WG, et al. Multifactorial risk index for predicting postoperative respiratory failure in men after major noncardiac surgery. The National Veterans Administration Surgical Quality Improvement Program. *Ann Surg*. 2000;232:242–253.

43. Brooks MJ, Sutton R, Sarin S. Comparison of Surgical Risk Score, POSSUM and p-POSSUM in higher-risk surgical patients. *Br J Surg*. 2005;92:1288–1292.

44. Collins TC, Daley J, Henderson WH, et al. Risk factors for prolonged length of stay after major elective surgery. *Ann Surg*. 1999;230:251–259.

45. Cockcroft DW, Gault MH. Prediction of creatinine clearance from serum creatinine. *Nephron*. 1976;16:31–41.

46. Guralnik JM, Ershler WB, Schrier SL, et al. J. Anemia in the elderly: a public health crisis in hematology. *Hematology Am Soc Hematol Educ Program*. 2005:528–532.

47. Steensma DP, Tefferi A. Anemia in the elderly: how should we define it, when does it matter, and what can be done? *Mayo Clin Proc* 2007;82:958–966.

48. Graeb C, Jauch KW. Surgery in immunocompromised patients. *Br J Surg*. 2008;95:1–3.

49. Dripps RD, Lamont A, Eckenhoff JE. The role of anesthesia in surgical mortality. *JAMA* 1961;178:261–266.

50. Collins TC, Johnson M, Daley J, et al. Preoperative risk factors for 30-day mortality after elective surgery for vascular disease in Department of Veterans Affairs hospitals: is race important?. *J Vasc Surg*. 2001;34:634–640.

51. Seshadri PA, Mamazza J, Schlachta CM, et al. Laparoscopic colorectal resection in octogenarians. *Surg Endosc*. 2001;15:802–805.

52. whqlibdoc.who.int/hq/2001/a73921.

53. Artz AS, Fergusson D, Drinka PJ, et al. Prevalence of anemia in skilled-nursing home residents. *Arch Gerontol Geriatr*. 2004;39:201–206.

54. Beghe C, Wilson A, Ershler WB. Prevalence and outcomes of anemia in geriatrics: a systematic review of the literature. *Am J Med*. 2004;116(Suppl 7A):3S–10S.

55. Kosmadakis N, Messaris E, Maris A, et al. Perioperative erythropoietin administration in patients with gastrointestinal tract cancer: prospective randomized double-blind study. *Ann Surg*. 2003;237:417–421.

56. Knight K, Wade S, Balducci L. Prevalence and outcomes of anemia in cancer: a systematic review of the literature. *Am J Med*. 2004;116 Suppl 7A: 11S–26S.

57. Davenport DL, Henderson WG, Khuri SF, et al. Preoperative risk factors and surgical complexity are more predictive of costs than postoperative complications: a case study using the National Surgical Quality Improvement Program (NSQIP) database. *Ann Surg*. 2005;242:463–468.

58. Bentrem DJ, Cohen ME, Hynes DM, et al. Identification of specific quality improvement opportunities for the elderly undergoing gastrointestinal surgery. *Arch Surg*. 2009;144:1013–1020.

59. Reiss R, Haddad M, Deutsch A, et al. Prognostic index: prediction of operative mortality in geriatric patients by use of stepwise logistic regression analysis. *World J Surg*. 1987;11:248–251.

60. Bender JS, Magnuson TH, Zenilman ME, et al. Outcome following colon surgery in the octagenarian. *Am Surg*. 1996;62:276–279.

61. Takeuchi K, Tsuzuki Y, Ando T, et al. Should patients over 85 years old be operated on for colorectal cancer? *J Clin Gastroenterol*. 2004;38:408–413.

62. Blair SL, Schwarz RE. Advanced age does not contribute to increased risks or poor outcome after major abdominal operations. *Am Surg*. 2001;67:1123–1127.

63. Bo M, Cacello E, Ghiggia F, et al. Predictive factors of clinical outcome in older surgical patients. *Arch Gerontol Geriatr*. 2007;44:215–224.

64. Cook TM, Day CJ. Hospital mortality after urgent and emergency laparotomy in patients aged 65 yr and over. Risk and prediction of risk using multiple logistic regression analysis. *Br J Anaesth*. 1998;80:776–781.

65. Loran DB, Hyde BR, Zwischenberger JB. Perioperative management of special populations: the geriatric patient. *Surg Clin North Am.* 2005;85:1259.

66. Lubin MF. Is age a risk factor for surgery? *Med Clin North Am.* 1993;77:327–333.

67. Eisenstaedt R, Penninx BW, Woodman RC. Anemia in the elderly: current understanding and emerging concepts. *Blood Rev.* 2006;20:213–226.

68. Wu WC, Schifftner TL, Henderson WG, et al. Preoperative hematocrit levels and postoperative outcomes in older patients undergoing noncardiac surgery. *JAMA.* 2007;297:2481–2488.

69. Moyes LH, Leitch EF, McKee RF, et al. Preoperative systemic inflammation predicts postoperative infectious complications in patients undergoing curative resection for colorectal cancer. *Br J Cancer.* 2009;100:1236–1239.

70. Al-Refaie WB, Parsons HM, Henderson WG, et al. Major cancer surgery in the elderly: results from the American College of Surgeons National Surgical Quality Improvement Program. *Ann Surg.* ;251:311–318.

71. McGory ML, Shekelle PG, Rubenstein LZ, et al. Developing quality indicators for elderly patients undergoing abdominal operations. *J Am Coll Surg.* 2005;201:870–883.

72. Lawrence VA, Hazuda HP, Cornell JE, et al. Functional independence after major abdominal surgery in the elderly. *J Am Coll Surg.* 2004;199:762–772.

73. Audisio RA, Gennari R, Sunouchi K, et al. Preoperative assessment of cancer in elderly patients: a pilot study. *Support Cancer Ther.* 2003;1:55–60.

74. Glasgow RE, Jackson HH, Neumayer L, et al. Pancreatic resection in Veterans Affairs and selected university medical centers: results of the patient safety in surgery study. *J Am Coll Surg.* 2007;204:1252–1260.

75. Dunne JR, Malone D, Tracy JK, et al. Perioperative anemia: an independent risk factor for infection, mortality, and resource utilization in surgery. *J Surg Res.* 2002;102:237–244.

76. Napolitano LM. Perioperative anemia. *Surg Clin North Am.* 2005;85(6):121527.

77. Wu WC, Smith TS, Henderson WG, et al. Operative blood loss, blood transfusion, and 30-day mortality in older patients after major noncardiac surgery. *Ann Surg.* 2010;252:11–17.

78. Silber JH, Rosenbaum PR, Trudeau ME, et al. Preoperative antibiotics and mortality in the elderly. *Ann Surg.* 2005;242:107–114.

79. Barlow AP, Zarifa Z, Shillito RG, et al. Surgery in a geriatric population. *Ann R Coll Surg Engl.* 1989;71:110–114.

80. Niv E, Elis A, Zissin R, et al. Abdominal computed tomography in the evaluation of patients with asymptomatic iron deficiency anemia: a prospective study. *Am J Med.* 2004;117:193–195.

81. Carsin AE, Sharp L, Cronin-Fenton DP, et al. Inequity in colorectal cancer treatment and outcomes: a population-based study. *Br J Cancer.* 2008;99:266–274.

82. Faragher IG, Chaitowitz IM, Stupart DA. Long-term results of palliative stenting or surgery for incurable obstructing colon cancer. *Colorectal Dis.* 2008;10:668–672.

83. Hanada K, Iiboshi T, Ishii Y. Endoscopic ultrasound-guided choledochoduodenostomy for palliative biliary drainage in cases with inoperable pancreas head carcinoma. *Dig Endosc.* 2009;21(Suppl 1):S75–S78.

84. Zauber AG, Lansdorp-Vogelaar I, Knudsen AB, et al. Evaluating test strategies for colorectal cancer screening: a decision analysis for the U.S. Preventive Services Task Force. *Ann Intern Med.* 2008;149:659–669.

85. Robinson TN, Eiseman B, Wallace JI, et al. Redefining geriatric preoperative assessment using frailty, disability and co-morbidity. *Ann Surg.* 2009;250:449–455.

86. Tran Ba Loc P, du Montcel ST, Duron JJ, et al. Elderly POSSUM, a dedicated score for prediction of mortality and morbidity after major colorectal surgery in older patients. *Br J Surg.* 2010;97:396–403.

87. Lloyd H, Ahmed I, Taylor S, et al. Index for predicting mortality in elderly surgical patients. *Br J Surg.* 2005;92:487–492.

88. Balducci L. Evidence-based management of cancer in the elderly. *Cancer Contl.* 2000;7:368–376.

Part 4: Data analysis
Dataset 1 analysed by Stata v11 (StataCorp LP, Texas, USA)

D1.1 Introduction

Postoperative dental pain is frequent after various forms of dental treatment, including orthodontic treatment to correct dental irregularities (malocclusions). Orthodontic treatment often involves the use of fixed appliances (braces) which, by using constant, gentle pressure, move teeth into their proper positions over a period of time. The two main components of the brace are the brackets that are placed on the teeth and the main archwire that connects them. At 'bond-up', the brackets are attached to the outer surface of the teeth with a special orthodontic bonding material. At the end of treatment, the brackets are 'de-bonded' (i.e. removed from the teeth).

Dr Angus Pringle kindly provided the data from a randomised controlled clinical trial to compare the effects on pain intensity for the 7 days after bond-up of two bracket (brace) types: the Tru Straight bracket (Ormco Europe, Amersfoort, The Netherlands) and the Damon 3 bracket (Ormco). The patients were each given a pain diary after bond-up, and they were asked to record their level of pain on 15 successive occasions using a visual analogue scale (VAS) at each time. The VAS was an unmarked horizontal 100 mm line, with 'no pain' at the left end of the line and 'extreme pain' at the right end. The patients recorded their perceived pain intensity levels before their evening meal on the day of bond-up and before breakfast and the evening meal for the next 7 days. At each time, the patients indicated whether they had consumed an analgesic over the intervening time period. On return of the questionnaire, the VAS scores were measured from the left margin of the line, providing a range of values of pain intensity from 0 to 100. The outcome measures were the maximum pain intensity over the period as well as the pain intensity on each occasion. The additional information collected from each patient comprised the baseline demographic characteristics (gender, age and ethnicity) and clinical characteristics (incisor class (I, II Division 1, II Division 2 and III), describing whether the upper or lower teeth were prominent, extraction or non-extraction treatment and three quantitative measures of the severity of contact point displacement (Little's Irregularity Index for the Lower Jaw, Little's Maxillary Irregularity Index for the Upper Jaw and Little's Total Irregularity Index, the third being the sum of the other two)).

A sample size calculation (Chapter 36) to determine the optimal number of patients required to demonstrate a difference of at least 20 on the VAS scale in maximum pain intensity between the two bracket groups with a standard deviation of 28.3 (obtained from a previously published study evaluating pain perception during orthodontic treatment with fixed appliances) indicated that 66 patients would be required in total. This calculation was based on an unpaired t-test with a power of 80% and a 5% level of significance.

Sixty-six patients entered the study, and 33 were randomly assigned to each bracket type. The questionnaires were not returned by five of the Tru Straight group and by nine of the Damon 3 group. No additional questionnaires were sent to the patients who failed to return them as they could not be completed retrospectively. Blinding of bracket allocation was impossible because the brackets were visible to both patient and orthodontist.

D1.2 Aims

The aims of this study were to assess whether the method of archwire ligation influenced pain intensity during the early stages (i.e. in the first week) of orthodontic treatment and to investigate the influence of age, ethnicity, gender, incisor class, extraction and severity of contact point displacement on pain intensity.

D1.3 Repeatability

In order to check that the repeatability of Little's Irregularity Index, Little's Maxillary Irregularity Index, Little's Total Irregularity Index and the VAS scores was acceptable, the measurements were repeated on 20 randomly selected individuals. For each measurement, a paired t-test was used to determine if there was a systematic difference, the limits of agreement were drawn in the Bland and Altman diagram, and the British Standards Institution repeatability coefficient and Lin's concordance correlation coefficients were determined. The paired t-tests did not show any evidence of a systematic difference ($P > 0.05$), the minimum value of Lin's concordance correlation coefficient was 0.98, suggesting good repeatability, and the Bland and Altman diagram showed no funnel effect in any instance, indicating that the repeatability was consistent whatever the magnitude of the measurement. Furthermore, the British Standards Institution repeatability coefficients were clinically acceptable.

To illustrate the procedures used, we summarise the results for Little's Total Irregularity Index. The paired t-test gave $P = 0.96$ with a mean difference of 0.010. The Bland and Altman diagram (Figure D1.1) showed the limits of agreement (−0.99 and 0.99) and demonstrated that the difference between the paired readings was constant through the range of values of the index. The standard deviation of the differences was 0.94 so that the British Standards Institution repeatability coefficient, representing the maximum likely difference between a pair of measurements, was approximately 1.88. Given that the mean of the measurements was 16.1, we believe that this is acceptable in terms of the error of measurement. Finally, Lin's concordance correlation

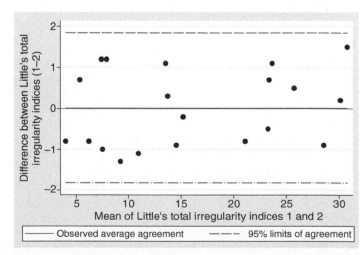

Figure D1.1 Bland and Altman diagram for Little's Total Irregularity Index.

Medical Statistics at a Glance Workbook, First Edition. Aviva Petrie and Caroline Sabin.
© 2013 Aviva Petrie and Caroline Sabin. Published 2013 by Blackwell Publishing Ltd.

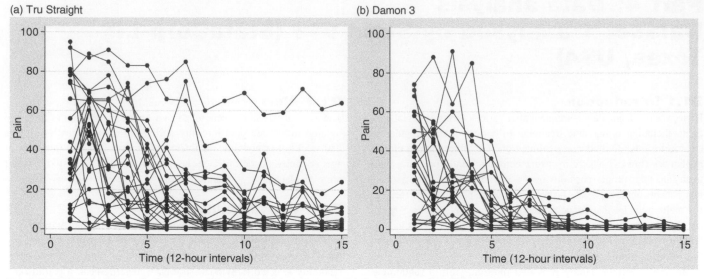

Figure D1.2 Pain on VAS scale for each patient at each 12-hour interval: (a) Tru Straight and (b) Damon 3.

coefficient was estimated as 0.96 (95% confidence interval (CI) 0.987 to 0.995).

D1.4 Getting a feel for the data

We show the pain intensity results on the VAS scale for each patient in Figure D1.2(a) for Tru Straight (coded 1), and in Figure D1.2(b) for Damon 3 (coded 2). Time 1 is before the evening meal on the day of bond-up (i.e. after the patients have been randomised and after they have received 'treatment'). Although it would be interesting to compare baseline pain values in the two groups, a patient does not suffer pain before the bracket is fitted, so baseline values are not measurable. Figure D1.3 shows the mean values in each group (with 95% CIs) at every 12-hour time point. There is a clear indication, when studying the latter graph in particular, that patients with the Damon 3 bracket experienced less pain intensity on average than those with the Tru Straight bracket, and the effect was similar at all times (i.e. there was no interaction between bracket type and time) apart from, perhaps, in the 12-hour interval from Time 1 = Day 1 before dinner to Time 2 = Day 2 before breakfast when the pain suffered by those on Damon 3 appeared to reduce substantially.

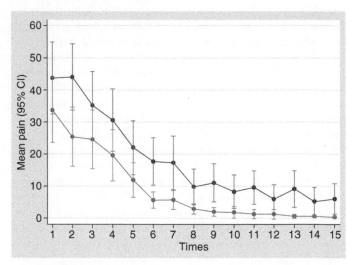

Figure D1.3 Mean pain at each time (95% CI) for Tru Straight (top line) and Damon 3 (bottom line). Time 1 = Day 1 before dinner, Time 2 = Day 2 before breakfast and each subsequent time is 12 hours later until Time 15 = Day 8 before dinner.

D1.5 Baseline data: comparability of bracket groups

Although randomisation was used, five patients in the Tru Straight and nine patients in the Damon 3 groups did not return their questionnaires, and this could have affected the comparability of the groups. In order to check this out, we drew a box plot and calculated the median, mean and standard deviation (SD) of each group for the numerical baseline variables (age and the three Little's irregularity indices). We assessed each categorical baseline variable (gender, incisor class, extraction and ethnicity) for group comparability by creating a contingency table and evaluating the proportions of patients in each group falling into the relevant categories. Because of the relatively large amount of missing data, we decided to perform significance tests (Chi-squared tests for categorical variables and unpaired *t*-tests or Mann–Whitney *U*-tests for numerical variables) to check for comparability of baseline variables, even

though we would not usually do this in a randomised trial. A significant result (using a significance level of 0.01 instead of the conventional 0.05 to avoid spuriously significant results arising from multiple testing) would suggest that bias might have been introduced by the omission of those patients who did not return their questionnaires.

Most of the variables were comparable in the two groups, but there was a significantly ($p < 0.001$) greater percentage of males fitted with the Tru Straight bracket (54%) than with the Damon 3 bracket (38%) and the incisor class distribution was not comparable ($p < 0.001$) with, for example, 36% of Tru Straight patients and only 25% of Damon 3 patients in Class 1. We noted, in addition, that the mean age of the patients fitted with the Tru Straight brackets (mean 16.11, SD 7.36 years) was slightly, but not significantly ($p = 0.08$), greater than that of those with the Damon 3 brackets (mean 15.21, SD 6.83 years).

Concern was therefore raised about the possible confounding effects (Chapter 34) of gender and/or incisor class on pain intensity, the outcome of interest. With this in mind, our approach was to adjust for any factor, including gender and incisor class, that could potentially confound the association between bracket type and pain intensity if we found that this factor was significantly associated with pain intensity (see Sections D1.6.2, D1.7.2 and D1.8.1).

D1.6 Maximum pain intensity analysis

Initially, we analysed the data by using a simple summary measures approach to deal with repeated measures data (Chapter 41). We began by considering only the maximum pain intensity suffered by the patient as this was of particular interest to the clinicians and the patients. We followed this by an area under the curve (AUC) analysis (Section D1.7).

D1.6.1 Univariable analyses of maximum pain intensity

We performed a series of univariable analyses to determine which, if any, of the baseline variables were associated with the maximum pain intensity experienced by the patients. For numerical baseline variables, this involved drawing a scatter diagram of maximum pain intensity against the variable and calculating and testing the Pearson correlation coefficient, r (Chapter 26), between the two variables. For categorical baseline variables and for bracket type, this involved drawing a box plot showing the distribution of maximum pain intensity in the different categories of the variable and performing an unpaired t-test or Mann–Whitney U-test (Chapter 21), or the Kruskal–Wallis test (Chapter 22), as appropriate. We set the significance level at 0.10 for the hypothesis tests performed (Chapter 33). We did not assess the effect of administering analgesia on maximum pain intensity as the application of analgesia is an intermediate variable that should not be treated as a confounder since it lies directly on the causal pathway (Chapter 34). However, we do discuss the effect of administering analgesia on pain intensity in the random effects regression analysis described in Section D1.8.

As an illustration of our findings, Figure D1.4 shows the distribution of maximum pain for each of the two bracket groups. The data in each group are approximately Normally distributed and so we performed an unpaired t-test, preceded by a variance ratio test (Chapter 35) to check for homogeneity of variance, to compare the mean maximum pain intensity in the two bracket groups. Box D1.1 contains the computer output from these analyses: $P = 0.96$ for the variance ratio test, indicating that there was no evidence of heterogeneity of variance, and $P = 0.04$ for the t-test, indicating that the mean maximum pain intensity suffered by patients with the Tru Straight bracket (mean 55.71, SD 4.77) was significantly greater than that with the Damon 3 bracket (mean 40.92, SD 5.08). The difference between the mean maximum pain intensities in the two groups was estimated as 14.80 (95% CI 0.78 to 28.81).

Using a 10% significance level, the only other variables that were statistically significantly associated with maximum pain intensity were extraction (with mean pain intensity being significantly greater (unpaired t-test, $P = 0.08$) in those patients with extraction (mean 57.88, SD 5.61) than in those with no extraction (mean 44.51, SD 4.46)) and Little's maxillary ($r = 0.34$, $P = 0.01$) and Little's total ($r = 0.29, P = 0.04$) irregularity indices. Since the former Little irregularity index is a component of the latter, only one of them (Little's Total Irregularity Index) was used in the multivariable regression analysis to avoid the problem of collinearity. However, we did also perform a sensitivity analysis by including Little's Maxillary Irregularity Index instead of Little's Total Irregularity Index as a covariate in the multiple regression analysis to see if this would affect the conclusions. Figure D1.5 is the matrix scatter diagram showing the relationship between maximum pain and each of Little's irregularity indices, demonstrating the type of illustration used for numerical variables.

D1.6.2 Multivariable linear regression analysis of maximum pain intensity

The next stage of the analysis was to perform a multivariable (multiple) linear regression analysis (Chapter 29), with maximum pain intensity as the outcome variable and bracket type (Tru Straight coded as 1 and Damon 3 coded as 2) as a covariate, together with those variables found to be statistically significant at the 10% level in the univariable analyses (i.e. extraction and Little's Total Irregularity Index). If gender and/or incisor class (the distribution of each was significantly different in the two bracket groups – see Section D1.5) had been significantly associated with maximum pain, we would have included them as additional covariates to avoid the problem of confounding. However, as neither demonstrated a significant relationship with maximum pain intensity, they were not included in the analysis.

The output for this regression analysis is shown in Box D1.2. We used a 5% significance level in the multivariable regression analysis. After adjusting for extraction and Little's Total Irregularity Index, the mean maximum pain intensity experienced by patients fitted with Damon 3 brackets was significantly less on average (difference in means 14.49, 95% CI 0.82 to 28.16, $P = 0.038$) than that of those fitted with the Tru Straight bracket. Neither of the other explanatory variables had a significant effect on maximum pain intensity, after adjusting for the effect of bracket type. Interestingly, the observed difference of 14.5 in the mean level of pain intensity experienced by the patients in the two bracket groups was less than the clinically relevant value of 20 used in the sample size calculation (Section D1.1). Thus, in spite of statistical significance, the result may not be clinically meaningful. However, we should be cautious when adopting this view as the upper limit of the 95% CI for the difference in means was 28.2 which would be regarded as clinically important.

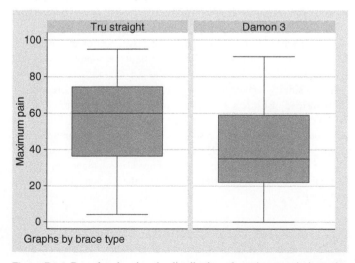

Figure D1.4 Box plot showing the distribution of maximum pain intensity in the two bracket groups.

Box D1.1 Variance ratio test and unpaired *t*-test comparing maximum pain intensity in the two groups

```
Variance ratio test
--------------------------------------------------------------------------
   Group |     Obs        Mean    Std. Err.   Std. Dev.   [95% Conf. Interval]
---------+----------------------------------------------------------------
Tru stra |      28    55.71429    4.768131    25.23058    45.93089    65.49768
 Damon 3 |      24    40.91667    5.084759    24.91013    30.39804    51.43529
---------+----------------------------------------------------------------
combined |      52    48.88462    3.595776    25.92951    41.66579    56.10344
--------------------------------------------------------------------------
        ratio = sd(Tru stra) / sd(Damon 3)                    f =    1.0259
Ho: ratio = 1                                degrees of freedom =    27, 23

     Ha: ratio < 1              Ha: ratio != 1              Ha: ratio > 1
  Pr(F < f) = 0.5208        2*Pr(F > f) = 0.9583          Pr(F > f) = 0.4792


Two-sample t test with equal variances
--------------------------------------------------------------------------
   Group |     Obs        Mean    Std. Err.   Std. Dev.   [95% Conf. Interval]
---------+----------------------------------------------------------------
Tru stra |      28    55.71429    4.768131    25.23058    45.93089    65.49768
 Damon 3 |      24    40.91667    5.084759    24.91013    30.39804    51.43529
---------+----------------------------------------------------------------
combined |      52    48.88462    3.595776    25.92951    41.66579    56.10344
---------+----------------------------------------------------------------
    diff |            14.79762    6.977635                 .782626    28.81261
--------------------------------------------------------------------------
     diff = mean(Tru stra) - mean(Damon 3)                    t =    2.1207
Ho: diff = 0                                 degrees of freedom =        50

     Ha: diff < 0                Ha: diff != 0               Ha: diff > 0
  Pr(T < t) = 0.9805        Pr(|T| > |t|) = 0.0389        Pr(T > t) = 0.0195
```

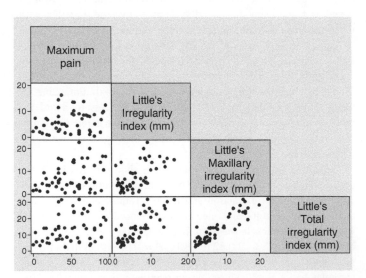

Figure D1.5 Matrix scatter diagram showing the relationship between maximum pain intensity and each of Little's irregularity indices.

Note that the difference in means obtained from the regression analysis was very similar to that obtained in the univariable analysis (i.e. 14.80, 95% CI 0.78 to 28.81), which is hardly surprising given that the other covariates in the model were not found to be independently associated with maximum pain intensity.

In order to check the assumptions underlying the regression analysis (Chapter 29), we applied some post-estimation commands in Stata to save the residuals and predicted values from the model. We then plotted the residuals against the predicted values to check for homoscedascity, and the residuals against each of the explanatory variables to check the linearity assumption. These assumptions appeared to be satisfied since there was a random scatter of points with no funnel effect in Figure D1.6(a) and no obvious relationship between the residuals and each of the covariates: as an illustration, we show the residuals plotted against Little's Total Irregularity Index in Figure D1.6(b). In addition, a histogram of the residuals (Figure D1.6(c)) indicated that the Normality assumption was not of concern.

A sensitivity analysis, using Little's Maxillary Irregularity Index instead of Little's Total Irregularity Index as a covariate in the multiple regression analysis (see Section D1.6.1), did not substantially change the results (difference in maximum pain means = 13.77, 95% CI 0.23 to 27.31, $P = 0.046$). Our conclusion, that the maximum pain intensity experienced by a patient was significantly lower on average for those fitted with the Damon 3 bracket, was unaltered.

D1.7 AUC of pain intensity analysis
We performed an additional summary measures analysis by considering the area under the curve (AUC) for each patient (Chapter 41).

Box D1.2 Output from the multivariable regression analysis for maximum pain intensity

```
      Source |       SS       df       MS              Number of obs =      52
-------------+----------------------------             F(  3,     48) =    3.21
       Model | 5730.11563        3  1910.03854         Prob > F      =  0.0311
    Residual | 28559.1921       48  594.983168         R-squared     =  0.1671
-------------+----------------------------             Adj R-squared =  0.1151
       Total | 34289.3077       51  672.339367         Root MSE      =  24.392


-------------------------------------------------------------------------------
 Maximumpain |     Coef.   Std. Err.      t    P>|t|     [95% Conf. Interval]
-------------+-----------------------------------------------------------------
  Littletotal |  .6262028   .5421066     1.16   0.254    -.4637756    1.716181
   Extraction |  6.165671   9.648086     0.64   0.526    -13.23311    25.56445
    Bracetype | -14.48784   6.798104    -2.13   0.038    -28.15635   -.8193399
        _cons |  59.52951  12.21664      4.87   0.000     34.9663    84.09271
-------------------------------------------------------------------------------
```

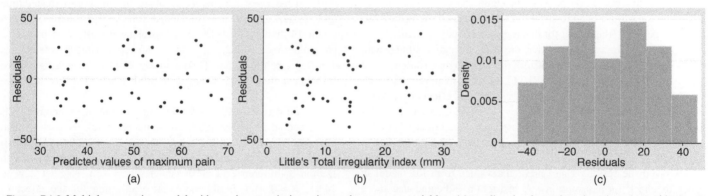

(a) (b) (c)

Figure D1.6 Multiple regression model with maximum pain intensity as the outcome variables: (a) predicted values plotted against the residuals; (b) scatter matrix showing the relationship between the residuals and Little's Total Irregularity Index and (c) histogram of the residuals.

We felt that this variable provided a useful summary of the level of pain suffered by a patient over the whole 7 days. If we consider the pain intensity on the VAS experienced by a single patient and connect the pain intensities at all the successive time points (see Figure D1.2), we obtain a pain 'curve' for that patient. We determined the AUC by dividing the total area under the 'curve' into a number of rectangles (area = base × height) and triangles (area = ½ base × height) and summed their areas. We analysed these AUCs in the same way that we analysed the maximum value of pain intensity in Section D1.6. We summarise our findings briefly.

D1.7.1 Univariable analysis of AUC

Initially, we performed a series of univariable analyses (Mann–Whitney or Kruskal–Wallis tests and tests for the Pearson correlation coefficient) to determine which, if any, of the baseline variables were associated with the AUC for pain intensity.

As an illustration of our findings, Figure D1.7 shows the distribution of AUC for each of the two bracket groups. The AUC for pain intensity was significantly greater ($P = 0.01$) in the Tru Straight group (median 171.1, range 10–989) than in the Damon

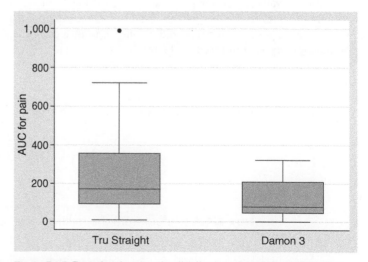

Figure D1.7 Box plot showing the distribution of AUC for pain in the two bracket groups.

3 group (median 79.3, range 0–322). The only other variables that were significant at the 10% level were gender, with males having a significantly ($P = 0.09$) greater AUC for pain on average (median 177.8, range 10–721.5) than females (median 109.8, range 0–989), and age, for which the Pearson correlation coefficient, estimated at 0.39 (95% CI 0.13 to 0.60), was significantly different from zero ($P = 0.004$).

D1.7.2 Multivariable linear regression analysis of AUC

We then performed a multivariable (multiple) linear regression analysis (Chapter 29), with the AUC for pain intensity as the outcome variable and bracket type (Tru Straight coded as 1 and Damon 3 coded as 2) as a covariate, together with those variables found to be statistically significant at the 10% level in the univariable analyses (i.e. gender and age). Gender was one of the variables that we found had a significant association with bracket type in Section D1.5 and that raised concerns about confounding. Incisor class, the other variable highlighted in Section D1.5, was not significantly associated with AUC and so we did not include it as a covariate in the model. We show an extract of the output for this regression analysis in Box D1.3. After adjusting for age and gender, the AUC for patients fitted with the Damon 3 bracket was significantly less on average (difference in means = 116.7, 95% CI 22.7 to 210.6) than that of those fitted with the Tru Straight bracket. Only age had a significant effect on the AUC, with the AUC increasing on average by 9.6 (95% CI 3.1 to 16.1) for a one year increase in age, after adjusting for the effect of bracket type and gender. Gender was not a significant ($P = 0.50$) covariate in the model.

We saved the residuals and predicted values from the model in order to check its assumptions. A histogram indicated that these residuals were approximately Normally distributed. We were not concerned about the linearity assumption when we observed the scatter of points after plotting the residuals against each of the explanatory variables. However, there was a suggestion that homoscedasticity might be present when we plotted the residuals against the predicted values, and this might have affected the P-values. A multiple linear regression analysis on various transformations of the AUC values (e.g. the square root) did nothing to resolve this issue. We therefore decided to revert to the original multivariable regression model and, because none of the P-values for the coefficients in the regression model was close to the significance level of 0.05, concluded that patients fitted with the Damon 3 bracket had a significantly lower AUC for pain on average than those fitted with the Tru Straight bracket.

D1.8 Random effects analysis of longitudinal data

D1.8.1 Random effects analysis with time as a series of dummy variables

We used a random effects model (Chapter 42) which recognised the longitudinal nature of the data to analyse the full data set using pain intensity at each assessment as the outcome variable.

We decided which explanatory variables to include in the final model by initially performing a series of random effects analyses, in each instance taking one of the baseline variables as the sole explanatory variable. With a significance level of 10%, the only significant baseline variable was age: for each additional year of age, the pain increased on average by 0.70 (95% CI 0.23 to 1.17, $P = 0.003$). Since neither gender nor incisor class (Section D1.5) was significantly associated with pain, we did not include them as covariates in the final model.

We then performed a random effects regression analysis with brace type and age as the explanatory variables. In addition, we treated time as a categorical variable and included it in the regression model as a set of 14 dummy variables, each assessing the effect on pain of a particular time i ($i = 2, 3, \ldots 15$) compared to Time 1 (where Time 1 = Day 1 before dinner, Time 2 = Day 2 before breakfast and each subsequent time is 12 hours later until Time 15 = Day 8 before dinner).

Box D1.4 contains the computer output from this random effects regression analysis. Using a 5% significance level, we can see that, after adjusting for the effect of age, patients with Tru Straight experienced significantly more pain intensity on average than those with Damon 3 (difference in mean pain levels = 8.63, 95% CI 2.34 to 14.91, $P = 0.007$). Furthermore, after adjusting for the effect of bracket type, older patients experienced a significantly greater level of pain on average than younger patients (for each additional year of age, the mean pain intensity increased by 0.66, 95% CI 0.22 to 1.10, $P = 0.003$). The mean pain intensity at every time, apart from that at Time 2, was significantly lower than that at Time 1, after adjusting for the other covariates in the model. The intra-class correlation coefficient, indicated by 'rho', was estimated as 0.46, indicating that 46% of the variation in pain intensity was explained by the differences between patients. Together with a highly significant result from the likelihood ratio test for clustering ($P < 0.001$), this confirmed the necessity to recognise the clustered nature of the data. We also noted when we looked at the coefficients in the output that there appeared to be a possible quadratic effect of time: this is also apparent from Figure D1.3.

Box D1.3 Output from the multivariable regression analysis for AUC of pain intensity

```
------------------------------------------------------------------------
     AUC |     Coef.   Std. Err.      t    P>|t|    [95% Conf. Interval]
---------+--------------------------------------------------------------
     Age |  9.636383   3.229073     2.98   0.004    3.143898    16.12887
  Gender | -32.00393   46.65977    -0.69   0.496   -125.8197    61.81182
Bracetype| -116.6506   46.73915    -2.50   0.016    -210.626   -22.67523
    cons |  258.8167   108.9225     2.38   0.022    39.81339    477.8201
------------------------------------------------------------------------
```

Box D1.4 Output from the random effects regression model with dummy variables for time

```
Fitting constant-only model:
Iteration 0:    log likelihood = -3497.8275
Iteration 1:    log likelihood = -3406.8727
Iteration 2:    log likelihood = -3386.5287
Iteration 3:    log likelihood = -3384.7784
Iteration 4:    log likelihood = -3384.7581

Fitting full model:
Iteration 0:    log likelihood = -3109.3739
Iteration 1:    log likelihood = -3109.0351
Iteration 2:    log likelihood = -3109.0339

Random-effects ML regression          Number of obs      =        780
Group variable: Patient               Number of groups   =         52

Random effects u_i ~ Gaussian         Obs per group: min =         15
                                                     avg =       15.0
                                                     max =         15
                                      LR chi2(16)        =     551.45
Log likelihood  = -3109.0339          Prob > chi2        =     0.0000


Pain          Coef.     Std. Err.       z       P>z      [95% Conf. Interval]

Age         .6607076    .2244728      2.94     0.003     .2207489    1.100666
Bracetype  -8.626785    3.207797     -2.69     0.007    -14.91395   -2.339618

Time
   2       -3.653846    2.339843     -1.56     0.118    -8.239853     .932161
   3       -8.788462    2.339843     -3.76     0.000    -13.37447   -4.202454
   4      -13.57692     2.339843     -5.80     0.000    -18.16293   -8.990916
   5      -21.75        2.339843     -9.30     0.000    -26.33601  -17.16399
   6      -26.98077     2.339843    -11.53     0.000    -31.56678  -22.39476
   7      -27.17308     2.339843    -11.61     0.000    -31.75908  -22.58707
   8      -32.5         2.339843    -13.89     0.000    -37.08601  -27.91399
   9      -32.26923     2.339843    -13.79     0.000    -36.85524  -27.68322
  10      -33.82692     2.339843    -14.46     0.000    -38.41293  -29.24092
  11      -33.36538     2.339843    -14.26     0.000    -37.95139  -28.77938
  12      -35.30769     2.339843    -15.09     0.000     -39.8937  -30.72169
  13      -33.96154     2.339843    -14.51     0.000    -38.54755  -29.37553
  14      -36.03846     2.339843    -15.40     0.000    -40.62447  -31.45245
  15      -35.69231     2.339843    -15.25     0.000    -40.27831   31.1063

_cons     41.3365      6.447311      6.41     0.000     28.70001    53.973

/sigma_u  11.08883     1.171482                         9.014884    13.63989
/sigma_e  11.93095      .3126728                        11.33359    12.55979
rho        .4634663     .0543747                         .3594355    .5700723

Likelihood-ratio test of sigma_u=0: chibar2(01)= 348.58 Prob>=chibar2 = 0.000
```

D1.8.2 Random effects model with time as a continuous variable

In view of the apparent quadratic nature of pain intensity over time, we performed a random effects regression analysis with brace type, age, time and time squared as covariates. We show the Stata output for this model in Box D1.5. All the covariates were significant at the 5% level. Using this approach, the difference in mean pain intensity experienced by those on Tru Straight compared to those on Damon 3 was almost identical to that obtained from the model using dummy variables for time (Section D18.1).

Although, after inspecting Figure D1.2, we did not expect a significant interaction between time and brace type (there is a difference in Time 1 values between the two brace types but, after that, they tend to decline at the same rate), we performed a further random effects analysis with the interaction terms of (brace type with time) and (brace type with time squared) as covariates in addition to brace type, time and time squared. Neither interaction term was significant ($P = 0.44$ and $P = 0.95$, respectively).

Finally, just as an exercise, we performed a random effects analysis with analgesia as a covariate in addition to time, time squared, age and brace type. As analgesia is on the causal pathway, we would have expected the inclusion of this variable in the model to attenuate the effect of brace type on pain, and this is exactly what we observed. The effect of analgesia was highly significant

($P < 0.001$), and the difference in mean pain intensity experienced by the two brace types was now lowered to 7.54 (95% CI 1.88 to 13.21, $P = 0.007$). However, we should emphasise that the effect of brace type can no longer be thought of as a causal effect in this model as we have adjusted for a factor that is on the causal pathway.

Finally, in order the check the assumptions underlying the model with time as a continuous variable and brace type, age, time and time squared as covariates, we used Stata post-estimation commands to save the predicted values and the between-patient (u) and within-patient (e) residuals from the model. Both the within- and between-patient residuals were approximately Normally distributed. There was a slight suggestion of homoscedasticity when the within-patient residuals were plotted against the predicted values as there tended to be greater variability in the between-patient residuals with increasing predicted values. Since there was some concern about the assumptions underlying the model, we performed a random effects regression analysis taking various transformations (e.g. square and fourth root of pain: logarithms were not appropriate as some pain intensities were zero) with brace type, age, time and time squared as covariates. The conclusions derived from the results were similar to those from the analysis that had pain intensity as the outcome variable, as were the diagrams used to check out the assumptions. Given that the effect of brace type in the model with pain as the outcome of interest was so marked

($P = 0.007$), we decided that, in spite of the fact that the homoscedasticity assumption could be regarded as questionable, overall the pain experienced by patients fitted with Tru Straight was significantly greater on average than that experienced by those fitted with Damon 3, and this effect was reasonably consistent over the 7-day period of the investigation.

D1.9 Summary

We analysed the data in various ways. We considered a summary measures approach, using, firstly, maximum pain and then the AUC as the outcome variable. We also analysed the data more comprehensively by using the levels of pain intensity at all 15 time points in a random effects regression analysis which recognised the clustered nature of the data. From the analyses, we concluded that patients fitted with the Damon 3 bracket experienced less maximum pain intensity and a lower level of pain on average than those fitted with the Tru Straight bracket. We did not find that there was a significant interaction of bracket type with time: the pain suffered by patients fitted with the two brackets declined at a similar rate over time. Finally, age was found to have a significant effect on the level of pain experienced by patients when the pain intensities were considered at all 15 time points and after adjusting for the effect of bracket type. This was apparent both in the multivariate regression analysis with AUC as the outcome variable and in the random effects regression analysis with pain intensity as the outcome variable: older patients tended to experience more pain than younger patients.

D1.10 Note
Further details of the randomised trial may be obtained from Pringle *et al.* (2009). In this publication, the results of an analysis of covariance are presented instead of the random effects model for the investigation of the effect of bracket type on the levels of pain intensity experienced by patients over time.

Reference

Pringle AM, Petrie A, Cunningham SJ, McKnight M. Prospective randomized clinical trial to compare pain levels associated with 2 orthodontic fixed bracket systems. Am J Orthod Dentofacial Orthop 2009; 136: 160–7.

Dataset 2 analysed using IBM SPSS Statistics v20

D2.1 Introduction

Hyposmia (a reduced ability to smell and detect odours) is a common finding in Parkinson's disease (PD). Two tests which evaluate the ability to smell different odours are the 40-item University of Pennsylvania Smell Identification Test (UPSIT-40) and the 16-item smell identification test from Sniffin' Sticks (SS-16). The UPSIT-40 smell identification test comprises four 'scratch-and-sniff' booklets that can be either self-administered or administered by a carer, nurse practitioner or physician. An individual is asked to identify the correct odour from four choices for every one of the 40 items, each being scored as 1 (correct identification of odour) or 0 (incorrect). The maximum UPSIT-40 score is therefore 40. Sniffin' Sticks uses scented felt-tip pens which are presented in sequence: the patient is asked to sniff the tip and identify the correct odour from four possible choices, each being scored as 1 (correct) or 0 (incorrect). The maximum score is therefore 16.

Dr Laura Silveira-Moriyama kindly provided data on a study she had performed to develop a clinical tool to simplify the interpretation of smell tests and facilitate their incorporation into the routine diagnosis of tremor disorders (Silveira-Moriyama *et al.*, 2009). She applied the UPSIT-40 and/or the SS-16 to 193 nondemented PD patients (diagnosed using clinical operational criteria for the diagnosis of PD combined with the intuitive clinical acumen of a movement disorder specialist) and 157 controls (recruited from among the staff and visitors to the same hospitals in the United Kingdom as the PD patients). The mean (standard deviation (SD)) of duration of PD was 10.2 (6.1) years and the mean age at onset of PD was 53.3 (10.3) years. These subjects had been group matched for age, gender and smoking habits, each of which can potentially influence the result of the smell test. In this current investigation, we evaluated the results of the two smell tests that had *both* been administered to a subgroup of 145 subjects: 89 PD and 56 controls. Information was collected on the subject's age at onset of PD (years), duration of PD (years), age (years), gender (female = 1, male = 2) and current smoking status (no = 0, yes = 1).

D2.2 Aims

The aims of our investigation were to compare the results from UPSIT-40 and SS-16 when used on PD patients and controls to determine the optimal tool for use in the routine diagnosis of Parkinson's disease and to evaluate the properties of this test as a diagnostic tool.

D2.3 Relationship between UPSIT-40 and SS-16

D2.3.1 Individual items of UPSIT-40 and SS-16

The individual odour items assessed in UPSIT-40 and SS-16 are shown in Table D2.1. All the SS-16 items were replicated by UPSIT-40 apart from garlic, coffee, apple, anise and fish. We calculated kappa values (Chapter 39) for the remaining 11 items. Interestingly, we found that the agreement between the two smell tests was not very good with kappa ranging from 0.14 (pineapple) to 0.46 (cloves) (i.e. from slight to moderate according to the Landis and Koch (1977) categorisations). This was not an unexpected finding, as the ability to correctly identify each item in such tests depends on the smell presented as much as on the alternatives for the forced choice. Although the smells presented were similar, the choices varied considerably between the tests, and this probably explains the poor agreement.

D2.3.2 Total scores of UPSIT-40 and SS-16

We investigated the relationship between the total scores of UPSIT-40 and SS-16 for an individual by drawing a scatter diagram (Figure D2.1) and calculating the Pearson correlation coefficient

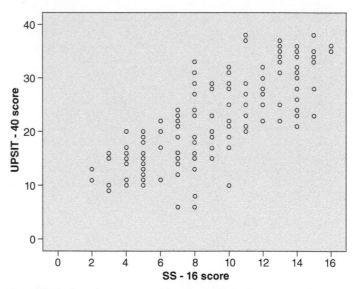

Figure D2.1 Scatter diagram showing the relationship between UPSIT-40 and SS-16 scores.

Table D2.1 Individual items (shown in the order in which they were presented) in the UPSIT-40 and SS-16 smell tests

UPSIT-40					SS-16	
Pizza	Leather	Strawberry	Dill pickle	Smoke	Orange	Garlic
Bubble gum	Coconut	Cedar	Pineapple	Pine	Leather	Coffee
Menthol	Onion	Chocolate	Lime	Grape	Cinnamon	Apple
Cherry	Fruit punch	Gingerbread	Orange	Lemon	Peppermint	Cloves
Motor oil	Liquorice	Lilac	Wintergreen	Soap	Banana	Pineapple
Mint	Cheddar cheese	Turpentine	Watermelon	Gas	Lemon	Rose
Banana	Cinnamon	Peach	Paint thinner	Rose	Liquorice	Anise
Love	Gasoline	Root beer	Grass	Peanut	Turpentine	Fish

Medical Statistics at a Glance Workbook, First Edition. Aviva Petrie and Caroline Sabin.

70   © 2013 Aviva Petrie and Caroline Sabin. Published 2013 by Blackwell Publishing Ltd.

($r = 0.80$, 95% confidence interval (CI) 0.73 to 0.85, $P < 0.001$). Thus, although the agreement was not very good between the individual items of the smell tests when considering only those items that were common to both tests, there was a highly significant relationship between the two tests when their total scores were evaluated, demonstrating that both tests probably measure the same thing: the overall ability to identify odours.

Note

All the analyses which follow use the total UPSIT- 40 and the total SS-16 scores for an individual. For simplicity we omit the term 'total' when referring to them and commonly use the abbreviated versions, UPSIT and SS.

D2.4 Univariable analyses

We were primarily interested in determining whether the total scores from each of the smell tests were significantly ($P < 0.10$) associated with disease status (PD or control). However, as age, gender and current smoking status are known to be distributed differently in those with and without PD, we were concerned that these variables should not be overlooked.

Although the original group of 350 patients and controls had been group matched for age, gender and current smoking status, we used only a subset of the group for our analysis (i.e. those individuals who had been given both smell tests). To check that the PD and control groups were still comparable with respect to them, we performed a two-sample *t*-test to compare the mean ages (Chapter 21) and Fisher's exact test (Chapter 24) to compare the distribution of gender and of current smoking status in the two groups. The box plot (Chapter 4) showed that age was approximately Normally distributed in each group: the mean (SD) age of the 89 PD and 56 control individuals was 62.82 (9.10) years and 64.36 (9.89) years, respectively ($P = 0.35$). Thirty eight (42.7%) of the PD patients and 21 (37.5%) of the control individuals were females ($P = 0.33$). Four (4.7%) of the PD patients and 2 (4.0%) of the controls were current smokers ($P = 0.61$) (note: three PD patients and six control subjects did not provide information about current smoking status). Thus, in spite of including only a subset from the original study, the group matching element was maintained, with age, gender and current smoking status appearing to be similarly distributed in the PD and control groups. This precluded the possibility of assessing the effects of these variables on PD, but this, in any case, was not the objective of the current study.

We then examined the distributions of UPSIT and SS in PD patients and controls by drawing box plots (Figure D2.2 (a) and (b)), generating summary measures of the test scores (Box D2.1) and comparing the mean values in the two groups for each test by performing a two-sample *t*-test (Chapter 21), after checking for homoscedasticity by Levene's test (Chapter 35). The difference in the mean scores (95% CI) was 11.03 (8.85 to 13.21) for UPSIT and 5.68 (4.81 to 6.56) for SS, with $P < 0.001$ for each test.

D2.5 Logistic regression analyses

D2.5.1 Logistic regression analyses to assess the effectiveness of UPSIT and SS to predict disease status

Our intention was to perform a multivariable logistic regression analysis (Chapter 30) with disease status (PD patient coded as 1 and control individual coded as 0) as the outcome variable and using any variables significantly associated with disease status in the univariable analyses as the explanatory variables. Our primary interest was in determining the effectiveness of UPSIT and SS in predicting disease status. However, since they were the only variables significantly associated with disease status in the univariable analyses (a not unexpected finding since the group matching for age, gender and current smoking status has been maintained in our subset of subjects), there were no other explanatory variables to include in the logistic regression analysis

In order to determine whether UPSIT or SS was the better predictor of PD, we initially performed a separate logistic analysis

---

Box D2.1 SPSS output showing summary statistics for UPSIT and SS scores in the two groups

	Diagnosis	N	Mean	Std. Deviation	Std. Error Mean
UPSIT score	Control	56	29.41	6.030	.806
	PD	89	18.38	6.714	.712
SS score	Control	56	12.66	2.193	.293
	PD	89	6.98	2.812	.298

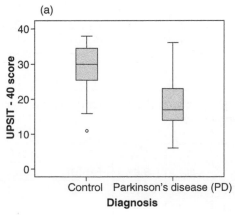

(a)

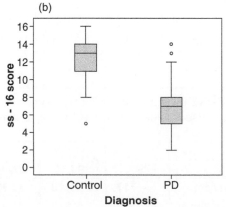

(b)

Figure D2.2 Box plot showing the distributions of (a) UPSIT-40 and (b) SS-16.

for each smell test, rather than including both of them as covariates in a multivariable model. We decided to do this because of the highly significant correlation between UPSIT and SS scores and the concern that including them as two covariates in an extended model might lead to collinearity (Chapter 33). Note that performing separate logistic regression analyses for each smell test would be expected to produce the same results as those obtained when simply performing unpaired t-tests to compare the mean UPSIT and SS scores in the two groups. However, because we also intended to perform a multivariable logistic regression analysis with both UPSIT and SS as explanatory variables, and because we hoped to be able to use the appropriate logistic regression model to predict the probability that a patient with a known smell test score had PD, we proceeded with the separate logistic regression analyses.

To facilitate a direct comparison of the partial regression coefficients from the two logistic models (recognising that the scales were different with the potential maximum score being 40 for UPSIT and 16 for SS), we standardised each UPSIT and SS score to obtain a Z score by subtracting the relevant mean (22.64 for UPSIT, 9.17 for SS) and dividing by the relevant standard deviation (8.40 for UPSIT, 3.79 for SS). The estimated partial regression coefficients for the smell tests for these models were -1.92 (95% CI -2.51 to -1.33, $P < 0.001$) for the standardised UPSIT and -2.72 (95% CI -4.54 to -1.90), $P < 0.001$) for the standardised SS. This suggested that although both smell tests were highly significant predictors of the log odds of being a PD patient, the SS association was somewhat stronger than the UPSIT association. When the exponential of each partial regression coefficient was taken (obtaining estimated odds ratios of 0.15 (95% CI 0.08 to 0.27) for the standardised UPSIT score and 0.07 (95% CI 0.03 to 0.15) for the standardised SS score), the odds of having PD was reduced by 85% (95% CI 73% to 92%) for a unit increase in the standardised UPSIT score and by 93% (95% CI 85% to 97%) for a unit increase in the standardised SS score.

We then performed a multivariable logistic regression analysis with the standardised UPSIT and standardised SS scores as covariates. The results are shown in Box D2.2, where 'Sig' in SPSS represents the P-value and a value of 0.000 for it implies $P < 0.001$. In this model, the effect of UPSIT on disease outcome was not statistically significantly different from zero ($P = 0.27$) after adjusting for the effect of SS, although the effect of SS remained highly significant ($P < 0.001$) after adjusting for the effect of UPSIT. Thus, it would appear that SS is a better predictor of PD than UPSIT. In spite of our original concerns that this model might be affected by collinearity, the standard errors of the estimated coefficients were not unduly large (extremely large standard errors may indicate collinearity) and one of the coefficients was significant (collinearity, in the presence of large standard errors, may be indicated if neither coefficient is significant in the multivariable model but each is significant in the relevant univariable model).

D2.5.2 Deriving the logistic regression equation and using it for prediction

We used the results from a logistic regression analysis to evaluate the probability that a particular patient had PD from his or her SS or UPSIT score. As explained in Section D2.5.1, we came to the conclusion that SS, rather than UPSIT, was probably the optimal tool for use in the routine diagnosis of Parkinson's disease in a group of individuals such as those included in this investigation. Consequently, for simplicity, we limit our explanations in this section to only SS.

To be able to predict the probability that an individual with a particular SS score has PD, we performed a logistic regression analysis with disease status as the outcome variable and SS score as the explanatory variable. We did not use standardised scores here as we required a tool that could be universally used and easily understood. Box D2.3 shows the estimated regression coefficients from this logistic regression model. The -2 log likelihood (i.e. the deviance or model Chi-square), equal to 93.54 on 143 degrees of freedom, was highly significant with $P < 0.001$ indicating that the coefficient of SS in the model was significantly different from zero (as confirmed by the Wald test statistic and

Box D2.2 SPSS output of the logistic regression analysis with disease status as the outcome variable and standardised UPSIT and SS scores as covariates

	B	S.E.	Wald	df	Sig.	Exp(B)	95% C.I.for EXP(B)	
							Lower	Upper
ZSSscore	−2.357	.510	21.322	1	.000	.095	.035	.258
ZUPSITscore	−.450	.405	1.231	1	.267	.638	.288	1.412
Constant	1.079	.304	12.611	1	.000	2.940		

Box D2.3 SPSS output of the logistic regression analysis with disease status as the outcome variable and unstandardised values of SS as the explanatory variable

	B	S.E.	Wald	df	Sig.	Exp(B)	95% C.I.for EXP(B)	
							Lower	Upper
SSscore	−.717	.110	42.320	1	.000	.488	.393	.606
Constant	7.636	1.179	41.953	1	.000	2071.5		

Table D2.2 Contingency table showing the number of subjects with and without PD according to the true diagnosis and the decision rule SS ≤ 10

	True diagnosis		Total
	Control	PD	
SS > 10 (not PD)	45	10	55
SS ≤ 10 (PD)	11	79	90
Total	56	89	145

Sensitivity = 79/89 = 0.89 (95% CI 0.82 to 0.95); specificity = 45/56 = 0.80 (95% CI 0.70 to 0.91); positive predictive value = 79/90 = 0.88 (95% CI 0.81 to 0.95) and negative predictive value = 45/55 = 0.82 (95% CI 0.72 to 0.92).

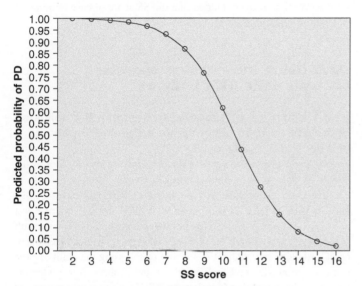

Figure D2.3 Predicted probability of PD from the logistic regression model plotted against SS score.

P-value in Table D2.2). The estimated logistic regression equation was logit p_{PD} = $\log_e p_{PD} / (1 - p_{PD})$ = 7.64 − 0.72SS, where p_{PD} is the probability of PD for an individual. The exponential of the regression coefficient for SS represents an estimated odds ratio. Thus, as the SS increased by one, the odds of having PD decreased by approximately 51% (95% CI 49% to 61%).

The odds ratio and *P*-value from this model provide evidence that the SS score is a useful predictor of PD but neither is particularly helpful if the clinician wants to have an idea of how likely it is that a presenting patient, with a known SS score, has PD. One way of achieving this is to substitute the SS value into the logistic regression equation provided in the previous paragraph. For example, if p_{PD} represents the probability that a patient has PD and the patient has an SS score of 5, then $\log_e (p_{PD} / (1 - p_{PD}))$ = 7.65 − 0.72 × 5 = 4.05. Hence $p_{PD} / (1 - p_{PD})$ = exp(4.05) = 57.40 and therefore p_{PD} = 0.98. Thus, this patient with an SS score of 5 has a 98% chance of having PD.

To get an idea of how the probability of having PD changes with the SS score, we saved the predicted values from the model and plotted them against the SS scores (Figure D2.3). It is clear that the probability of PD increases with decreasing SS score (i.e. when the sense of smell declines). With this diagram, the clinician can easily assess the likelihood of PD in a subject with a particular SS score. For example, if a subject has an SS score of 10, his or her chance of having PD is just

over 60%, whereas if the subject's SS score is 11, the chance of PD is just under 45%.

D2.5.3 Using the logistic regression equation to provide a decision rule

We also used the logistic model to determine a cut-off for SS which provided a decision rule for the diagnosis of PD. We wanted to choose a cut-off so that if a subject had an SS score equal to or below it, he or she was more likely to have PD than not have it. In this case, the probability of PD would be more than 0.5. If required, we could have modified the approach by choosing a different probability (e.g. 0.6). When we substituted p_{PD} = 0.5 into the logistic regression equation, we found that:

$\log_e (0.5 / (1 - 0.5))$ = 7.64 − 0.72 × SS, and so
SS = (7.64 − log1) / 0.72 = (7.64 − 0.00) / 0.72 = 10.6

(note that this value is approximate as we rounded the values of the coefficients). Hence, if a patient had an SS score of 10 or below (recognising that SS can take integer values only), that patient was more likely to have PD than not have it. Table D2.2 is a two-way contingency table showing the number of subjects who did or did not have PD according to the true diagnosis and the decision rule (using a threshold of SS = 10).

We evaluated the effectiveness of this diagnostic test by considering its sensitivity and specificity, and its usefulness by evaluating its positive (PPV) and negative (NPV) predictive values (Chapter 38), as shown in the footnote of Table D2.2. The relatively high values of these indices certainly suggest that an SS score of 10 or lower provides an effective and useful diagnostic test for PD in individuals such as those in our investigation.

D2.5.4 Logistic regression model assumptions and diagnostics

If the results from the logistic regression analysis are to be viewed with confidence, it is important to check the underlying assumptions of the model and run some model diagnostics which might identify outliers and influential points (Chapters 30 and 35).

a) *Extra-binomial dispersion.* We checked for extra-binomial dispersion by dividing the deviance (i.e. the likelihood ratio statistic (LRS), also denoted by −2log likelihood (−2LL)) by 143 (i.e. the sample size minus 2). The deviance = 93.541 was obtained from the SPSS output, and the quotient was therefore equal to 93.541 / 143 = 0.7. There did not appear to be evidence of extra-binomial dispersion since the ratio was not substantially less (or greater) than one.

b) *Goodness of fit.* The Hosmer–Lemeshow test gave Chi-squared = 6.22, with degrees of freedom = 7 and P = 0.52. This non-significant result indicated that there was no evidence that the model was a poor fit.

c) *Checking for linearity.* To check the linearity assumption (Chapter 33), we categorised the subjects into five equally sized subgroups (based on the quintiles of SS), calculated the log odds of PD for each subgroup and plotted the log odds of PD against the midpoint of the range of values of SS for the corresponding subgroup (Figure D2.4). The linear pattern exhibited by the log odds values in the subgroups suggested that the linearity assumption of the logistic model was satisfied.

d) *Logistic regression diagnostics.* We saved the standardised (normalised) and deviance residuals, leverage and DfBeta values from the model with a view to identifying outliers and influential points.

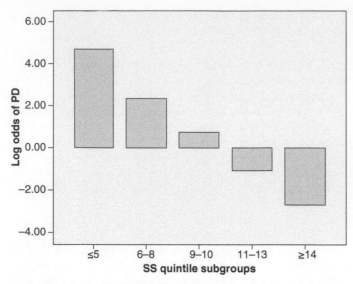

Figure D2.4 Log odds of PD plotted against the midpoint of the each quintile subgroup of SS to check for linearity.

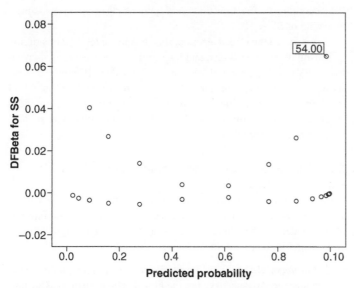

Figure D2.5 DFBeta plotted against predicted probability of PD.

We plotted each of these against both the predicted values and the case numbers. From a number of these graphs, it was apparent that case number 54 might be an influential point: Figure D2.5 shows one of these graphs with case number 54 highlighted.

Case number 54 was a 76-year-old nonsmoking control subject with SS = 5, so he would have been classified incorrectly as a PD patient using an SS score of 10 or lower to indicate PD. On discussions with Dr Laura Silveira-Moriyama, the clinician who was leading the investigation and familiar with the clinical manifestations of each patient, it was decided this man could have a biologically plausible result. He might have had smell problems from other diseases that were not ruled out by the exclusion criteria. There are many causes of problems with smell which cannot be accounted for in the clinical screening process (e.g. a viral infection such as flu or the common cold which can cause permanent smell loss). Because it would artificially improve the accuracy of the method, we decided it was not sensible to exclude a control who was misclassified as a PD patient unless his or her score was lower than 4 (such scores

would be lower than that expected by chance alone). We decided, however, that it would be of interest to determine whether case number 54's SS score was influential by repeating the analysis excluding this case. When we excluded case number 54, we obtained logit $p = 8.48 - 0.79SS$ as the estimated logistic regression equation. This was very similar to the equation obtained on the full data set when the estimated regression coefficient for SS was 0.72. There was no change in the P-value for this coefficient ($P < 0.001$) or in the cut-off for SS to diagnose PD which was 10.7 instead of 10.6, both implying that SS should be ≤ 10 to diagnose PD in a subject. There was very little difference in the sensitivity and specificity with values of 88.8% and 81.8%, respectively, instead of 88.8% and 80.4% from the model based on the data set which included this subject. We therefore concluded that the SS score of case number 54 was not an influential point.

D2.6 Using the receiver operator characteristic (ROC) curves

D2.6.1 Using the ROC curves to compare the abilities of the two tests to discriminate between PD patients and controls

The nonparametric ROC curve (Chapter 38) is a two-way plot of the sensitivity against one minus the specificity for different cut-offs of the diagnostic test of interest. We plotted the ROC curves for UPSIT and SS (Figure D2.6), every point on a curve for a particular test allowing us to compare the probabilities of a positive smell test result in those with and without PD. We calculated the area under each curve (AUC, AUROC or c-statistic) as a way of assessing the ability of the test to discriminate between PD patients and controls. A test which is perfect at discriminating between the two disease categories has the c-statistic $= 1$, and a nondiscriminatory test which performs no better than chance has the c-statistic $= 0.5$. We estimated the c-statistics in this study as 0.89 (95% CI 0.82 to 0.94) and 0.93 (95% CI 0.89 to 0.97) for UPSIT and SS, respectively, suggesting that both tests were good but SS was the probably the better smell test overall. However, it should be noted that the ROC curves do not take account of the fact that the results of the smell tests are paired (i.e. each subject used both SS and UPSIT) and so any comparison of the ROC curves should be viewed with caution.

D2.6.2 Using the ROC to determine an optimal cut-off for diagnosing PD

Since the c-statistics and the results of the logistic regression analyses (Sections D2.5) suggested that SS, rather than UPSIT, was likely to be the optimal tool for use in the routine diagnosis of Parkinson's disease in a group of individuals such as those studied, we concentrate in this section on SS for simplicity.

Using logistic regression (Section D2.5.3), we determined that if a subject had an SS score equal to or below the threshold of 10, then that subject was more likely (with a probability exceeding 0.5) to have PD than not have it. This approach assumed that the 'cost' of a false positive diagnosis (i.e. an individual who was incorrectly diagnosed with PD) was equivalent to that of a false negative diagnosis (i.e. a PD patient who was incorrectly diagnosed as not having PD); equivalently, it assumed that the sensitivity and specificity of the test had equal importance. Very often we wish, instead, to choose that threshold for a diagnostic test which provides

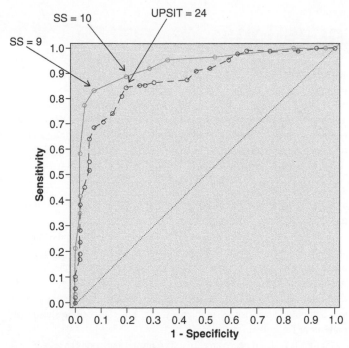

Figure D2.6 ROC curves for SS score (solid line) and UPSIT score (dashed line) with dotted reference line.

Table D2.3 Sensitivity, specificity and likelihood ratio for PD for different SS score thresholds with PD indicated if SS ≤ cut-off

SS cut-off	Sensitivity	Specificity	Likelihood ratio (SS ≤ cut-off)
1	0.000	1.00	–
2	0.034	1.00	–
3	0.090	1.00	–
4	0.213	1.00	–
5	0.348	0.982	19.3
6	0.416	0.982	23.1
7	0.584	0.982	32.4
8	0.775	0.964	21.5
9	0.831	0.929	11.7
10	0.888	0.804	4.5
11	0.921	0.714	3.2
12	0.955	0.643	2.7
13	0.966	0.464	1.8
14	1.000	0.161	1.6
15	1.000	0.036	1.0
16	1.000	0.000	–

the optimal combination of sensitivity and specificity that satisfies the particular requirements of the test (e.g. it might be more desirable for a test to have a high sensitivity rather than a high specificity, or vice versa). If we wish to use the ROC curve to choose the threshold, treating the sensitivity and specificity as equally important, the optimal cut-off will be that value of the test score corresponding to the point on the ROC curve nearest the top left-hand corner of the graph: Zweig and Campbell (1993) suggest a technique for determining that point as it is not always obvious when eyeballing the diagram. In the SS ROC curve in Figure D2.6, the point in the top left corner is that for which the sensitivity = 0.83 and the specificity = 0.93, corresponding to a cut-off for the SS score of 9. In this study, however, we believed that the sensitivity was more important than the specificity because we were more interested in being able to assess whether a subject has PD rather than whether he or she did not have it. We therefore chose a threshold which provided a greater sensitivity without unduly compromising the specificity. In particular, we regarded the optimal threshold for the SS score to be that point in Figure D2.6 for which the sensitivity = 0.89 and the specificity = 0.80, and this corresponded to a SS score cut-off of 10 (shown in Figure D2.6).

We also assessed these thresholds by evaluating the likelihood ratios (LR) for PD: the LR is equal to the sensitivity / (1 minus specificity) and it describes how much more likely the subject is to have PD than not have it for a particular cut-off (Chapter 38). Table D2.3 lists the different values of the sensitivity, specificity and likelihood ratio for PD for various SS score thresholds. The greatest likelihood ratio of PD (32.4) corresponded to SS ≤ 7 with sensitivity = 0.58 and specificity = 0.98. However, we felt that this was not satisfactory because the sensitivity was so low. The threshold of SS = 10 (equal to that determined by logistic regression analysis) gave a likelihood ratio for PD of 4.5. Thus an individual would be nearly five times more likely to have PD than be a control if his

or her SS score was less than or equal to 10. An individual with any SS score of less than 10 would be even more likely to have PD than be a control (i.e. the LR for PD was 11.4 for SS ≤ 9 and between 19.3 and 32.4 for SS ≤ 8), but these cut-off values had slightly lower or very much lower sensitivities. It may be of interest to note that when using an UPSIT score threshold of 24 (chosen from the optimal combination of sensitivity (0.84) and specificity (0.80): see Figure D2.6), the likelihood ratio for PD = 4.3, so an individual would be more than four times more likely to have PD than be a control if his or her UPSIT score was less than or equal to 24.

D2.7 Conclusion

After considering all the results obtained from our analysis, we decided that an SS score of less than or equal to 10 provided an acceptable diagnostic test for PD in a group of subjects similar to those used in our investigation. We should remember that these subjects came from a larger group of PD patients and controls who were originally group-matched for age, gender and current smoking status, and we found that these variables were similarly distributed in the PD patient and control groups in our subset. Thus it was not feasible to assess the effects of these variables on PD. Ideally we should assess this diagnostic tool for generalisablity by testing it on a different group of individuals, preferably those whose characteristics are more representative of the population of PD patients and controls.

References

Landis JR, Koch GG. *The measurement of observer agreement for categorical data. Biometrics 1977; 33: 159–74.*

Silveira-Moriyama L, Petrie A, Williams DR, Evans A, Katzenschlager R, Barbosa ER, Lees AJ. *The use of a color coded probability scale to interpret smell tests in suspected Parkinsonism. Mov Disord 2009; 24(8): 1144–53.*

Zweig MH, Campbell G. *Receiver-operating characteristic (ROC) plots: a fundamental evaluation tool in clinical medicine. Clin Chem 1993; 30(4): 561–77.*

Part 5: Solutions
Solutions to multiple-choice questions

M1

a) False: As the variable can take only whole numerical values, it is best described as a discrete variable.

b) False: Important information may be lost if only the final total score is recorded on the data capture form. It is preferable to record the scores for each task separately; the total score can then be calculated from them.

c) True: Although this is strictly an ordinal categorical variable, it may be possible to treat this variable as a numerical variable for the purposes of analysis.

d) False: Although it would be possible to calculate the modal value for this variable, given the large number of categories, it would be preferable to treat this variable as a numerical variable and calculate the median or, possibly, the mean score.

e) False: Whilst this approach may ultimately be useful, at this stage we have no indication of the number of individuals whose scores fall into each of these three categories (and thus whether these categories are the most 'sensible' for analytical purposes). Furthermore, by categorising the variable in this way, we are discarding potentially useful information.

M2

a) False: A qualitative variable comprises two or more categories which may be ordinal or nominal rather than numerical.

b) False: An ordinal variable comprises categories which are ordered. A nominal variable comprises categories which cannot be ordered.

c) False: The age groups 'young', 'middle aged' and 'old' relate to an ordinal categorical variable.

d) True: Blood group is classified as a nominal categorical variable.

e) False: It may be difficult to distinguish a discrete numerical variable from an ordinal variable when the ordinal variable has many categories.

M3

a) False: Although some statistical packages would recognise that a blank entry represents a 'missing' data value, this is not true for all packages. Furthermore, it is difficult to know whether a blank cell represents a truly missing value (i.e. the information is not available) or whether the person completing the questionnaire has simply forgotten to complete the entry. Thus, where possible, it would be preferable to allocate a code for a missing value at the design stage.

b) False: By only recording the data in categories in this way, important information may be lost about the number of eggs consumed.

c) False: It is feasible that some adolescents may actually consume nine eggs in a week – thus, with a code of 9 for a missing value, it will be difficult to distinguish between these adolescents and those for whom the data are missing.

d) False: By only recording the data in categories in this way, important information may be lost about the number of eggs consumed. Furthermore, as no code is provided for a missing value, it is difficult to distinguish between genuinely missing data and simple errors in data entry.

e) True: This approach captures the full information about the number of eggs consumed over the week. In addition, there is no potential confusion between a missing value and either a genuine entry or a data entry error.

M4

a) False: Having data available as an ASCII file is flexible because it can be read by most packages.

b) False: A multi-coded question has more than two possible responses, and more than one answer is possible for each respondent.

c) False: Dates may be entered into a computer spreadsheet in many ways, but the format should be consistent for a given data set.

d) False: Missing data for a particular respondent may be entered on the computer spreadsheet in many ways, but the format should be consistent for a given data set.

e) True: It is often necessary to assign numerical codes to a categorical variable before entering the data into the computer.

M5

a) False: Although it is true that the entry of 71 is an outlier, it is unlikely that this would be a correct value of weekly egg consumption and the authors should investigate this further.

b) False: The authors should investigate all potential outlying values before taking appropriate measures to deal with them, for example by using analytical methods that are not affected by outliers (such as the use of transformations or nonparametric tests) or by repeating the analysis with and without the outlying values to assess the impact of their exclusion on the results. Outliers should not be routinely excluded; further investigation is warranted.

c) False: The authors should investigate all potential outlying values before taking appropriate measures to deal with them, for example by using analytical methods that are not affected by outliers (such as the use of transformations or nonparametric tests) or by repeating the analysis with and without the outlying values to assess the impact of their exclusion on the results. Routine replacement of outlying values with values that are thought to be closer to those 'expected' is not usually recommended.

d) False: Although it is possible that 71 is an error, the authors should not automatically replace its value without investigating the potential error in more detail.

e) True: This is one appropriate method of dealing with outlying values in a data set; other appropriate methods may include the use of transformations or nonparametric tests.

M6

a) True: One approach to handling outliers in a data set is to analyse the data both with and without the outliers and see whether the results are similar.

b) False: In some instances, it may be sensible to transform data to overcome the problem of a skewed distribution in order to satisfy the assumptions underlying the proposed statistical techniques.

Medical Statistics at a Glance Workbook, First Edition. Aviva Petrie and Caroline Sabin.

Although it is often difficult to meaningfully interpret the parameter estimates obtained from the transformed data, depending on what the transformation entails, interpretation may be straightforward after back-transformation.

c) False: Outliers in data should not be omitted from the analysis *automatically* even if they skew the results. Depending on the proposed statistical analysis, measures may be taken to deal with outliers, such as taking transformations, using nonparametric techniques or, in some instances, performing the analysis both with and without the outliers.

d) False: An outlier is an extreme value which is incompatible with the main body of the data. However, it is sometimes greater and sometimes less than the main body of the data.

e) False: In addition to dealing with outliers by analysing the data both with and without the outliers to determine the effect of the omission, omitting the outlier(s) from the analysis or transforming the data, nonparametric methods are often used.

M7

a) **True**: A bar chart is useful for displaying discrete data with a limited range of values and categorical data.

b) False: A histogram is useful for displaying continuous data; as the number of eggs consumed in a week is a discrete numerical variable, a bar or column chart would be preferable.

c) False: A pie chart is most useful for displaying variables that are categorical with few categories. The number of eggs consumed in a week is a discrete numerical variable, and a bar chart would be preferable.

d) False: A scatter diagram is most useful for displaying the association between two variables. As we have only a single variable to display, a scatter diagram would not be feasible.

e) False: A segmented bar chart is most useful for displaying the association between two categorical variables. As we have only a single variable to display, a nonsegmented bar chart would be more appropriate.

M8

a) **True**: By eye-balling the data, we can see that the distribution of values has a long tail to the right (i.e. it is skewed to the right).

b) False: By eye-balling the data, we can see that the distribution of values has a long tail to the right, and hence this distribution is skewed to the right rather than Normal.

c) False: By eye-balling the data, we can see that the distribution of values has a long tail to the right, and hence this distribution is skewed to the right rather than skewed to the left.

d) False: By eye-balling the data, we can see that the distribution of values has a long tail to the right, and hence this distribution is skewed to the right rather than uniformly distributed.

e) False: By eye-balling the data, we can see that the distribution of values has a long tail to the right, and hence this distribution is skewed to the right (positively skewed) rather than skewed to the left (negatively skewed).

M9

a) False: A pie chart is one in which a circular 'pie' is split into sectors, one for each category of a categorical variable, so that the area of each sector is proportional to the frequency in that category.

b) False: A sensible way of displaying continuous numerical data is to draw a histogram rather than a bar chart: the latter should be used for categorical data.

c) False: A histogram is a chart in which separate vertical (or horizontal) bars are drawn with no gaps between the bars, the width (height) of each bar relating to a specific range of values of the variable with its area proportional to the associated frequency of observations.

d) **True**: The distribution of a variable is right skewed if a histogram of observed values has a long tail to the right with one or a few high values.

e) False: A box-and-whisker plot comprises a vertical or horizontal rectangle indicating the interquartile range, within which is the median; the ends of the 'whiskers' often indicate minimum and maximum values but may relate to particular percentiles.

M10

a) False: As this variable is a discrete numeric variable, and eyeballing the data suggests that their distribution is skewed to the right, the arithmetic mean would not be a suitable measure of the 'average' value and the range would be unduly influenced by the extreme value of 71.

b) **True**: As this variable is a discrete numeric variable, and eyeballing the data suggests that their distribution is skewed to the right, the median and interquartile range would be appropriate summary measures.

c) False: As this variable is a discrete numerical variable, and eyeballing the data suggests that their distribution is skewed to the right, the median would be an appropriate measure of the 'average' value. Whilst the range might in some circumstances be used to display the spread of values, its upper limit would be heavily distorted by the extreme value of 71. By focusing on the central 50% of values, the interquartile range would be less affected by any extreme value and is preferable.

d) False: As this variable is a discrete numerical variable, and eyeballing the data suggests that their distribution is skewed to the right, neither the arithmetic mean nor the standard deviation would be suitable summary measures.

e) False: As this variable is a discrete numerical variable with a wide range of values, the mode would not be the optimal summary measure. Furthermore, the mode, by itself, provides no indication of the spread of the data values. Therefore, it would not be the preferred way of summarising the data.

M11

a) False: The median is greater than the arithmetic mean if the data are skewed to the left.

b) **True**: The median value of n observations is equal to the $(n + 1)/2^{th}$ value in the ordered set if n is odd.

c) False: The arithmetic mean and the weighted mean are always identical if the weights used in the calculation of the weighted mean are equal.

d) False: The logarithmic transformation of right-skewed data will often produce a symmetrical distribution when the transformed data are plotted on an arithmetic scale.

e) False: The geometric mean of a data set is equal to the anti-log of the arithmetic mean of the log-transformed data.

M12

a) False: The percentile method should be used only to generate reference ranges when the number of healthy individuals in the study is reasonably large (in this case, 212 healthy individuals may be regarded as reasonably large).

b) False: The authors have generated their reference range based on data collected on healthy individuals. By definition, 2.5% of healthy individuals in the population are expected to have a value that is below the lower limit of the reference range.

c) False: Although the mean and standard deviation of the sample can be used to generate a reference range, this approach makes the assumption that the underlying distribution of haemoglobin levels in the population is Normal. As the authors have not provided data to demonstrate this, we cannot conclude that such a reference range would necessarily be more suitable.

d) False: Although individuals in the population with an underlying health condition that has an impact on haemoglobin levels are likely to have values that will fall outside the reference range, this is by no means a certainty, and some such individuals may have values that fall within the reference range.

e) True: Individuals in the population with an underlying health condition that has an impact on haemoglobin levels are likely to have values that will fall outside the reference range, although this is by no means a certainty, and some such individuals may have values that fall within the reference range.

M13

a) False: The interquartile range is the difference between the first and third quartiles, equivalent to the 25th and 75th percentiles, respectively.

b) True: The interdecile range contains the central 80% of the ordered observations.

c) False: The middle observation in ordered numerical data is the median if the number of observations is odd. If the number of observations is even, the median is usually taken as the arithmetic mean of the middle two observations. It is rarely exactly equal to the arithmetic mean.

d) False: The 50th percentile is equal to the second quartile (i.e. the median).

e) False: The first percentile is not always equal to the minimum value: it has 1% of the ordered observations below it.

M14

a) False: The mean and median of the Gaussian distribution are equal.

b) False: The Gaussian distribution is often called the Normal distribution, but its observations are not necessarily derived from healthy individuals.

c) False: The Standard Normal distribution has a mean equal to zero and a variance equal to one.

d) False: 95% of the observations following a Gaussian distribution lie between the mean $\pm$ 1.96 times the standard deviation.

e) True: Approximately 68% of the observations following a Gaussian distribution lie between the mean $\pm$ the standard deviation.

M15

a) False: A Binomial random variable is the observed number of successes in the situation where there are only two possible outcomes, success and failure. The count of the number of events that occur randomly and independently in time or space at some fixed average rate relates to a Poisson random variable.

b) False: There is only one parameter characterising the Poisson distribution and that is the mean (i.e. the average rate). The two parameters that characterise a Binomial distribution are the number of individuals in the sample (or repetitions of a trial) and the true probability of success for each individual (or in each trial).

c) False: The Chi-squared distribution is a continuous probability distribution based on a continuous random variable.

d) True: When the logarithm of observations which follow the Lognormal distribution are taken, the transformed observations follow the Normal distribution.

e) False: The Lognormal distribution is highly skewed to the right.

M16

a) False: Although the use of a nonparametric analytical method would be possible for this variable, it may not be optimal. This is because the options for performing multivariable nonparametric methods are limited. Thus, if feasible, a preferable option would be to transform the variable in some way so as to achieve Normality.

b) False: The logarithmic transformation is likely to be successful at achieving Normality when the underlying variable is skewed to the right; it will not result in a Normally distributed variable when the underlying data are skewed to the left.

c) True: Use of the square transformation may help to achieve Normality when the underlying data are skewed to the left.

d) False: Although use of the square transformation may help to achieve Normality when the underlying data are skewed to the left, this is not a certainty. Furthermore, the square transformation may not ensure that the other assumptions underlying a parametric analysis are met (e.g. adequate sample size and equal variances).

e) False: Categorisation of a variable results in a loss of information which should be avoided where possible. Prior to making a decision to categorise age at menopause for an analysis, the authors should investigate the association between age at menopause and any outcome of interest. Where the true association can be described by a linear (or log-linear) relationship, categorisation in this way may result in loss of power.

M17

a) True: The logistic transformation linearises a sigmoid curve.

b) False: The logistic transformation is generally applied to proportions, i.e. binary outcomes.

c) False: If a numerical variable, y, is skewed to the left, the distribution of $z = y^2$ is often approximately Normal.

d) False: If a numerical variable, y, is skewed to the right, $z = \log y$ is often approximately Normally distributed.

e) False: The square transformation has properties which are the reverse of those of the logarithmic transformation.

M18

a) False: The sampling distribution of the mean represents the distribution obtained by taking many repeated samples of a fixed size from the population of interest and calculating the mean from each sample. A plot of these means, such as a histogram, shows the sampling distribution of the means.

b) **True**: The sampling distribution of the mean has a mean which is an unbiased estimate of the true mean in the population.

c) False: The sampling distribution of the mean follows a Normal distribution provided the sample size is reasonably large, even if the underlying data are not Normally distributed.

d) False: The sampling distribution of the mean has a standard deviation which is equal to the standard error of the mean.

e) False: The sampling distribution of the mean can be drawn regardless of the sample size of the repeated samples.

M19

a) False: Although it is true that the best estimate of the mean height of the Thai female population will be provided by the mean height in the sample, it is unlikely that the mean height in the population will exactly equal that in the sample. The 95% confidence interval for the mean will provide a range within which it is likely that the true mean height will lie.

b) False: Calculation of mean height $\pm 1.96 \times$ SD would give an indication of the range within which 95% of the height values lie – it would not give any indication of the precision of the estimated mean. To obtain this information, the authors should calculate the 95% confidence interval for the mean height (i.e. mean $\pm 1.96 \times$ SEM).

c) False: Although the median may provide a reasonable summary of the 'average' height in the sample, the confidence interval for the median will not provide any information about the spread of the values.

d) **True**: If the heights are approximately Normally distributed, the range given by mean $\pm 1.96 \times$ SD will provide a description of the expected range within which most (95%) of the values in the population will lie.

e) False: To investigate whether the height values in their sample are Normally distributed, the investigators should calculate the range given by mean $\pm 1.96 \times$ SD; this range should contain approximately 95% of the sample data values. If this is not the case, this provides an indication that the data are not Normally distributed. Although it is possible to use the confidence interval for the mean to obtain an estimate of the standard deviation, this would require several additional calculations and would not be the preferred route.

M20

a) False: The outcome in this study is the percentage of patients who return to theatre with a wound complication within 30 days of initial surgery; as such, this is a binary outcome variable which is never Normally distributed.

b) False: If we were to repeat this experiment many times, the true wound complication rate would fall between 0.9% and 3.5% on 95% of occasions. However, there is a small chance that the true wound complication rate might fall outside this range.

c) False: Although the 95% confidence intervals for the true wound complication rates in the two periods overlap, it is not possible to conclude that there was no significant change in the wound complication rate. To formally test this, we would need to perform a significance test (e.g. a Chi-squared test) or evaluate the (95%) confidence interval for the difference in the wound complication rates and observe whether or not it contained zero.

d) False: The confidence interval for the percentage (for a given number of patients included in the denominator) is widest when the estimated percentage is close to 50; as the estimated percentage moves towards 0 or 100, the width of the confidence interval will be reduced. Thus, it is difficult to know whether the confidence interval would become wider without knowing the number of wound complications.

e) **True**: The main factor that determines the width of the confidence interval for a percentage is the number of individuals in the denominator; as this number increases, the width of the confidence interval decreases.

M21

a) False: The 99% confidence interval for the mean is wider than the 95% confidence interval for the mean.

b) **True**: The 95% confidence interval for the mean of a particular variable is narrower than the reference interval for that variable.

c) False: If the true standard deviation is known, the 95% confidence interval for the mean is calculated as the mean ± 1.96 times the standard error of the mean.

d) False: The 95% confidence interval for the mean broadly represents the interval within which the population mean falls with 95% certainty. The sample mean will always be contained in the confidence interval for the mean.

e) False: The 95% confidence interval for the mean broadly represents the interval which contains the population mean with 95% certainty.

M22

a) False: As there is an intervention involved, this study would be more accurately described as an experimental study.

b) **True**: As the medical students are followed over time without any interventions applied, this would be described as a cohort study.

c) False: As there is an intervention (regular counselling support), this is more accurately described as a clinical trial (albeit a nonrandomised one) rather than a cohort study (which is an observational study with no intervention).

d) False: As this study compares individuals who fail their end-of-first-year exams to a random sample of those who passed their end-of-first-year exams in terms of lifestyle factors over the previous year, this study would be described as a case–control study.

e) False: This type of study is an ecological cross-sectional study.

M23

a) False: The cause must precede the effect if causation is to be demonstrated.

b) False: The association between cause and effect should be assessed in an observational study on the basis of statistical results together with biological reasoning (i.e. the association should be plausible).

c) **True**: If feasible, then removing the potential causative factor of interest should reduce the risk of disease.

d) False: Although the larger the association between the cause and the effect, the more likely that it is causal, a small association can also mean that there is a causal effect.

e) False: It may be sufficient to imply causation on the basis of a single study if the association between the cause and effect in that study is strong and, particularly, if there is also a strong (and proven) biological mechanism to explain the relationship. However, it is *usually* insufficient to imply causation on the basis of the results from a single observational study: there should ideally be consistent results from a number of studies.

M24

a) False: The investigators chose a cross-over design as the appliances are unlikely to have a long-term impact on snoring symptoms. Cross-over designs are suitable only for interventions that do not have a long-lasting effect on the outcome.

b) False: The use of a cross-over design has no impact on the length of treatment time that is required – that should be determined on the basis of clinical need rather than on any statistical or design considerations.

c) False: In general, use of a cross-over design allows investigators to recruit a smaller number of participants rather than a greater number.

d) False: The washout period in a cross-over design is incorporated in order to allow any residual effects of the previous treatment to dissipate.

e) **True**: Using each participant as his or her own control is a benefit of the cross-over design, assuming that the treatment only temporarily relieves symptoms and does not provide a cure.

M25

a) False: Not being able to make a decision in advance is not a valid reason for the choice of an endpoint, which should be based on clinical opinion. A composite endpoint may be used in situations where there are several outcomes, each of which are deemed (in advance) to have clinical relevance.

b) False: The use of a composite endpoint does not, in general, simplify the analysis. If all components of the endpoint have equal clinical relevance, then the composite endpoint can be analysed as if it were a simple binary or time-to-event endpoint; if, however, some components of the endpoint are deemed to have greater clinical relevance than others, appropriate analytical methods that correctly incorporate this information should be used.

c) **True**: If one or more components of the composite endpoint are deemed to have greater clinical relevance than others, then appropriate analytical methods, which take this into consideration, must be used when analysing a trial that utilises a composite endpoint.

d) False: In general, follow-up of an individual in a trial might stop as soon as the person experiences one component of the endpoint, at which time he or she may be withdrawn from the trial – in many situations, therefore, information is not collected about the true frequency of each component, only on its frequency as the 'first' event that occurred.

e) False: One of the benefits of using a composite endpoint is that patients may experience an endpoint sooner than had the trial considered only one component of the endpoint. Thus, if anything, the length of the trial may be reduced, although this is by no means a certainty.

M26

a) False: A factorial design is one in which there is more than one factor of interest and these factors are analysed simultaneously.

b) False: A statistical interaction exists between two factors (e.g. drug treatments and drug doses) in a clinical trial when the difference between the levels or categories of one factor (e.g. treatments) is not the same for each level or category of the other factor (e.g. doses).

c) False: The cross-over trial in a clinical setting is an example of a within-individual comparison. If there are two treatments, each individual gets both treatments, one after the other in random order, with a washout period between them, and the difference in the responses on the two treatments for each individual is used to analyse the data.

d) False: A parallel trial comparing two treatments is one in which each individual receives only one of the treatments that are to be compared.

e) **True**: A complete randomised design is one in which the experimental units are assigned randomly to the treatments and there are no other refinements to the design.

M27

a) False: Using a cluster randomised trial to reduce the size of the trial is not a valid reason for choosing a cluster design. A cluster design would be chosen if it is felt it would not be feasible to randomise individual parents to an intervention (which is the case here, where the intervention would be applied at the school level).

b) False: A cluster randomised design was chosen as it was felt that it would be *impossible* to individually randomise the parents of each child to the intervention.

c) **True**: A cluster randomised design was chosen as it was felt that it would be impossible to treat the parents of each child in a school as independent units of investigation in the trial.

d) False: The unit of investigation for the trial is the school rather than the individual adult driving each car.

e) False: When calculating the sample size for this trial, the investigators must make allowance for the fact that the intervention is applied at the school level rather than the individual level. Usually the overall sample size (i.e. the number of parents) is greater in a cluster randomised trial than if a cluster design had not been used.

M28

a) False: The secondary endpoints in a clinical trial are those that are of less consequence than the primary endpoint which relates to the main aim of the study. The primary endpoint is usually concerned with treatment efficacy, whereas the secondary endpoints are often concerned with toxicity.

b) False: Randomisation of individuals to patients in a clinical trial is a process devised to avoid allocation bias. The main purpose is to promote similarity between the comparison groups so that any prognostic factors are evenly distributed in these groups and any differences in response can be attributed to treatment.

c) False: A sequential trial is one in which the patients enter the clinical trial serially in time, and the cumulative data are analysed as they become available by performing repeated significance tests. A decision is made after each test on whether to continue sampling or to stop the trial by rejecting or not the null hypothesis.

d) **True**: Blocked randomisation is used so as to achieve approximately equally sized groups at the end of patient recruitment in a clinical trial.

e) **False**: Systematic allocation is a method of allocating individuals to treatments in a clinical trial in a systematised, nonrandom manner. Systematic allocation includes alternating or using the last two digits of the year of birth.

M29

a) **False**: As the authors do not include any 'control' individuals who have not retired in their study, it will be difficult to fully quantify the effect of retirement on the incidence of depression in the population.

b) **False**: By restricting their analyses to the subgroup of participants who remain under follow-up for the full 5-year period, the authors may introduce selection bias, particularly if those who are lost to follow-up differ in any regard (particularly in terms of their incidence of depression) from those who remain in the study.

c) **False**: The primary outcome measure of the study is the incidence of depression over the 5-year period; this calculation must exclude any individuals who already had depression at the time of retirement, although calculation of the prevalence could include these individuals.

d) **True**: To ensure that retirement precedes any symptoms of depression, the study investigators should exclude any individual who already has depressive symptoms at recruitment from their calculation of the incidence of depression.

e) **False**: As the information on depressive symptoms will be collected prospectively, there cannot be any recall bias; this is a particular problem encountered in retrospective case–control studies where the quality of information on the exposure may be different in cases and controls.

M30

a) **False**: The time sequence of events can be assessed in a cohort study.

b) **True**: The cohort study can provide information on a wide range of disease outcomes.

c) **False**: It is not difficult to study exposure to factors that are rare in a cohort study.

d) **False**: The risk of disease can be measured directly in a cohort study.

e) **False**: A cohort study is generally expensive to perform.

M31

a) **False**: 32/816 would be the odds of tuberculosis (TB) in the sample of Moroccan immigrants in the Netherlands (number of individuals with TB divided by the number of individuals without TB); however, as this is a case–control study, and the number of cases and controls in the study are set as part of the study design, the odds of TB do not provide any meaningful interpretation in this setting.

b) **False**: 32/848 would be the prevalence of TB in the sample of Moroccan immigrants in the Netherlands (the number of individuals with TB divided by the total number of individuals in the sample); however, as this is a case–control study, and the number of cases and controls are set as part of the study design, the prevalence of TB does not have any meaningful interpretation in this setting.

c) **False**: The odds ratio for this study is 3.16 (= (26/6) ÷ (472/344)), which suggests that Moroccan immigrants in the Netherlands who travel to TB-endemic countries have more than a three times greater odds of experiencing TB than those who do not travel to TB-endemic countries. Note that 1.40 = 81/58 is the percentage of travellers to TB-endemic countries amongst those with TB divided by the percentage of travellers to TB-endemic countries amongst those without TB, indicating that there is a 40% increased risk of traveling to TB-endemic countries in those with TB compared to those without TB.

d) **False**: As this study is a case–control study, it is not possible to directly estimate the relative risk (as the number of cases and controls are set as part of the study design). However, when the outcome is rare (as is the case in this study), both the odds ratio and relative risk provide very similar information. In this situation, therefore, it is unlikely that different information would be gained by presenting the relative risk.

e) **True**: The odds ratio for this study is 3.16 (= (26/6) ÷ (472/344)), which suggests that Moroccan immigrants in the Netherlands who travel to TB-endemic countries are over three times more likely to experience TB than those who do not travel to TB-endemic countries.

M32

a) **True**: A case–control study is particularly suitable for rare diseases.

b) **False**: Loss to follow-up is not a common problem in a case–control study.

c) **False**: The relative risk cannot be used to estimate the effect of the exposure on the disease outcome in a case–control study as the starting point includes those with and without the disease, so the risk of disease in these groups is 1 and 0, respectively. The odds ratio is used instead of the relative risk.

d) **False**: The case–control study is an example of a retrospective observational study.

e) **False**: The case–control study is an example of an observational study rather than an experimental study because the investigator does not intervene in the care of the patient in any way in a case–control study.

M33

a) **True**: As the cases and controls in this study are individually matched, the authors should use conditional logistic regression to analyse the outcomes of the study.

b) **False**: If a variable is used as part of the matching process in a case–control study, it is no longer possible to analyse the impact of that particular variable on the outcome.

c) **False**: By ignoring the fact that the cases and controls are individually matched, the authors would reduce the power of their study.

d) **False**: Had the authors loosened their matching criteria to ensure that cases and controls were matched by age within 10 years rather than 5 years, it is likely that the results from the study would have been weakened as the matching process would have been less successful at removing the potentially confounding effect of age on the outcome.

e) False: As the cases and controls in this study are individually matched, and this is a case–control study, the authors should use conditional logistic regression to analyse the outcomes of the study. There is a binary outcome for each subject (i.e. with (a case) or without (a control) hepatocellular carcinoma), so multiple linear regression methods are not appropriate.

M34

a) False: If the hypothesised value for the effect of interest (e.g. the difference in means) in a hypothesis test lies within the 95% confidence interval for the effect, then this value is a plausible value for the effect and we do not have evidence to reject the hypothesis, $P > 0.05$.

b) False: A hypothesis test of superiority which proceeds by calculating a test statistic and relating it to the appropriate probability distribution to obtain the P-value is so called because we are usually interested in demonstrating that at least one treatment is better than (superior to) the other(s). The alternative may be an equivalence or a non-inferiority trial where interest is focussed on determining whether a new treatment is similar to or not substantially worse than existing treatments.

c) **True**: The test statistic that is calculated in a hypothesis testing procedure reflects the amount of evidence in the data against the null hypothesis.

d) False: A bioequivalence trial is a particular type of randomised trial in which we are interested in showing that the rate and extent of absorption of a new formulation of a drug are the same as those of an old formulation, when the two drugs are given at the same dose.

e) False: Nonparametric tests focus on drawing conclusions and making decisions (to reject or not reject the hypothesis under investigation). The information they provide does not include estimates of the effects of interest, and they contribute little by way of understanding the data.

M35

a) False: The authors used a Bonferroni correction to adjust their P-values to minimise the impact of multiple testing, introduced by the large number of laboratory markers that were considered as outcomes. By using this correction, the authors were less likely to obtain spuriously significant results.

b) False: The authors used a Bonferroni correction to adjust their P-values to minimise the impact of multiple testing, introduced by the large number of laboratory markers that were considered as outcomes.

c) False: The authors used a Bonferroni correction to adjust their P-values to minimise the impact of multiple testing, introduced by the large number of laboratory markers that were considered as outcomes.

d) False: Once a Bonferroni correction has been used to adjust the P-value from a study, the normal threshold for statistical significance (usually 0.05) should then be applied.

e) **True**: The authors used a Bonferroni correction to adjust their P-values to minimise the impact of multiple testing, introduced by the large number of laboratory markers that were considered as outcomes.

M36

a) False: The probability of making a Type I error is the chance of erroneously rejecting the null hypothesis. The power of the test is equal to one minus the probability of a Type II error.

b) **True**: The probability of making a Type I error is the probability of rejecting the null hypothesis when it is true.

c) False: The probability of making a Type I error is the probability of rejecting the null hypothesis when it is false. A Type II error is made when the null hypothesis is not rejected when it is false.

d) False: The probability of making a Type I error can never exceed 0.05 only if the significance level is set at 0.05.

e) False: The significance level of the hypothesis test is the maximum chance of making a Type I error.

M37

a) False: The authors chose to perform a one-sample t-test as they believed that the distribution of spleen length in the population was Normal.

b) False: The authors chose to perform a one-sample t-test as they wished to compare the mean spleen length in their population to a known population value.

c) False: We do not have any information on the distribution of spleen length in the population and so cannot conclude that it is likely to be highly skewed.

d) False: By including both men and women in the study, the authors aimed to answer a general question about spleen length among men and women in the population. If spleen sizes do not differ, on average, between men and women in the population, then it is possible that the results would be reliable. However, if spleen sizes do differ, the conclusions of this study would be unreliable if the gender composition in the authors' sample was very different from that in the population.

e) **True**: As the population mean value (8.94 cm) does not fall within the 95% confidence interval for the mean estimated spleen length, $P < 0.05$, this indicates significance at the 5% level.

M38

a) False: The one-sample t-test is used to test the null hypothesis that the population mean takes a particular value.

b) False: The assumption underlying the one-sample t-test is that the variable of interest follows a Normal distribution if the sample size is small. The test statistic then follows the t-distribution with degrees of freedom equal to the sample size minus one.

c) False: The sign test used on numerical data tests the null hypothesis that the number of values above (or below) the hypothesised value for the median is greater than one half.

d) **True**: The sign test used on numerical data evaluates the number of values in the sample that are greater (or less) than the median value specified in the null hypothesis and assesses whether it differs significantly from $n'/2$, where n' is the number of observations in the sample not equal to the specified median.

e) False: The sign test and one-sample t-test performed on the same set of numerical data will probably not give exactly the same P-value if the data are Normally distributed. Depending on whether the assumptions of the one-sample t-test are met, the conclusions drawn should be similar but the P-values are unlikely to be identical.

M39

a) False: As the two sets of results are not independent (i.e. the same individuals are assessed both pre- and post-intervention), a paired analysis should be performed to obtain maximum value from their data. As the two-sample t-test is not a paired test, this would not be optimal.

b) **True**: The outcome of interest in this study is the change in the number of correct answers after the intervention. Thus, the optimal summary measure would have been an indication of the average change in the number of correct answers from before to after the intervention, along with some indication of the spread of this. To choose the optimal summary measure, the authors should investigate the distribution of these changes and then select the mean or median as appropriate.

c) False: The Wilcoxon signed-ranks test is a nonparametric test that is appropriate for the analysis of paired data; the Wilcoxon rank-sum test or the Mann-Whitney U-test would be an appropriate choice of nonparametric test if the data sets were independent (i.e. if one group of individuals completed the questionnaire initially and a different group of individuals completed the questionnaire after the intervention).

d) False: The fact that the P-value is <0.05 suggests that the apparent improvement in knowledge is inconsistent with chance and is therefore likely to be a real finding.

e) False: Although the results of their study suggested that there was a significant increase in knowledge over the one-month period, the lack of a control sample (who did not receive the intervention) means that it is not possible to attribute this improvement to the intervention alone. It is possible that other changes may have occurred which could also have led to an improvement in knowledge, regardless of the intervention.

M40

a) False: The sign test can be used on numerical data. It can be used to test the null hypothesis that the median takes a particular value. It assesses whether the number of values in the sample above (or below) the hypothesised median is significantly different from $n'/2$, where n' is the number of observations in the sample not equal to the hypothesised median.

b) **True**: The Wilcoxon signed-ranks test is a more powerful test than the sign test when there are paired numerical observations. This is because it uses more information, that is, the actual values in the sample rather than the number of values above (or below) one half.

c) False: The Wilcoxon signed-ranks test is a nonparametric alternative to the paired t-test, not the other way around.

d) False: The two-sample t-test ignores the pairings in the data and so will not produce the same P-value as the paired t-test when there are two groups of paired numerical observations.

e) False: The assumption underlying the paired t-test is that, if the difference between each pair of readings is taken, these differences should be Normally distributed.

M41

a) False: As 'age group' has three categories, an unpaired t-test would not have been appropriate (it is useful only when comparing the means in two independent groups); a one-way analysis of variance (ANOVA) would have been a more appropriate choice of test.

b) **True**: As 'age group' has three categories, it would be appropriate to use a one-way ANOVA to investigate a possible association between the EPDS score and age group.

c) False: As both the Multidimensional Scale of Perceived Social Support (MSPSS) and the Edinburgh Postnatal Depression Scale (EPDS) are discrete numerical scores, it would not be appropriate to use an ANOVA to investigate the association between the two; a correlation coefficient (either Pearson's or Spearman's) would be a more appropriate choice of analysis.

d) False: The null hypothesis for the comparison would have been that there was no difference in the true mean EPDS score between the population of women who did receive health insurance and women who did not.

e) False: The paired t-test would be used when comparing the values of a single variable in two dependent groups. As the investigators are interested in investigating an association between two different variables (the MSPSS and the EPDS), a correlation coefficient (either Pearson's or Spearman's) would be a more appropriate choice of analysis.

M42

a) False: The Wilcoxon rank-sum test is a nonparametric alternative to the unpaired t-test.

b) False: The Wilcoxon signed-rank test cannot be performed if the two groups of observations are independent as the test relies on assessing the difference between paired observations. Hence it cannot produce the same P-value as the Mann Whitney U-test when comparing two groups of independent observations.

c) False: The null hypothesis for the unpaired t-test comparing two group means is that the population means are equal.

d) False: When the sample sizes are reasonably large, the unpaired t-test is reasonably robust to a departure from the underlying assumption of Normality in the two groups. It is not robust to a departure from the underlying assumption of equal variances.

e) **True**: When the sample sizes are reasonably large, the unpaired t-test is fairly robust to a departure from the assumption of Normality in each of the two groups.

M43

For the question concerning a one-way analysis of variance on three independent groups of numerical observations:

a) False: The null hypothesis is that the population means are all equal.

b) False: The null hypothesis is that the population means are all equal.

c) **True**: If the null hypothesis is rejected, then it can be concluded that at least one mean differs significantly from the others.

d) False: If the null hypothesis is rejected, then it can be concluded that there is a difference between at least two of the group means.

e) False: The sample sizes do not have to be the same in the three groups.

M44

a) False: Fisher's exact test can be used to compare the percentages in two groups only if the numbers experiencing and not experiencing the adverse event in each of the two groups are known. In this study, the numbers experiencing and not experiencing the adverse event are known in the experimental treatment group, but they are not provided for the general population. However, the percentage with the event in the general population is known, so the percentage of individuals who experienced the event in their study could be compared with the known percentage using a test statistic which relies on the exact Binomial test or on the Normal approximation to the Binomial distribution.

b) False: The (Wilcoxon) signed-ranks test is used when comparing numerical or ordinal data from two related groups. In this situation, the individuals in the experimental treatment group are not related to the individuals in the general population, so a paired analysis is not appropriate.

c) True: As the percentage with the event in the population is known, the percentage of individuals who experienced the event in the study could be compared with the known percentage using a test statistic which relies on the exact Binomial test or on the Normal approximation to the Binomial distribution.

d) False: The Chi-squared test can be used to compare percentages in two groups only if the numbers experiencing and not experiencing the adverse event in each of the two groups are known. In this study, the numbers experiencing and not experiencing the adverse event are known in the experimental treatment group, but they are not known in the general population.

e) False: McNemar's test can be used only when comparing two proportions between related groups. In this situation, the individuals in the experimental treatment group are not related to the individuals in the general population, so a paired analysis is not appropriate.

M45

a) False: The test statistic approximates the Normal distribution when the sample size is reasonably large.

b) True: A continuity correction should be applied to the test statistic if referring that test statistic to the Normal distribution to obtain a P-value.

c) False: If the 95% confidence interval for the true proportion excludes ½, the proportion is significantly different from ½, $P < 0.05$.

d) False: The data is binary categorical and so does not follow the Normal distribution.

e) False: (b) is true.

M46

a) False: To calculate the expected number of participants randomised to the dietary supplement with the primary endpoint, it is necessary to multiply 321 (the number randomised to this group) by 0.743 (= 474/638, the overall proportion that achieved the primary endpoint), not by 0.798 (the observed proportion with the primary endpoint in the dietary supplement group).

b) False: To calculate the expected number of participants randomised to the low-fat diet alone group with the primary endpoint, it is necessary to multiply 317 (the number randomised to this group) by 0.743 (= 474/638, the overall proportion that achieved the primary endpoint).

c) False: It is recommended that a continuity correction be applied to the Chi-squared test comparing two percentages, regardless of the size of the study.

d) True: As the important outcome of a Chi-squared test is simply a P-value, it is recommended that information is also provided on the treatment effect (e.g. the estimated difference in percentages in the two groups) as well as its associated 95% confidence interval.

e) False: As this is a randomised trial, there should be no confounding present (the patients are allocated to the treatment group at random, and so there should be no major systematic differences between the two groups). Thus, assuming that randomisation has been applied successfully, there should be no need to perform multivariable regression to remove the effects of any confounders. Furthermore, it should be noted that logistic regression is used when the outcome variable is binary: in this study, the outcome variable (weight loss) is numerical.

M47

a) False: The underlying assumption of the Chi-squared test to compare the two proportions is that the expected (not the observed) frequency in each of the four cells of the relevant contingency table should be at least five.

b) False: The underlying assumption of the Chi-squared test to compare the two proportions is that the expected frequency in each of the four cells of the relevant contingency table should be five or greater.

c) False: The expected frequency in a given cell of the contingency table is the frequency that would be expected in that cell if the true proportions were equal.

d) False: The Chi-squared test statistic should include a continuity correction because the data are not continuous.

e) True: The degree of freedom for the Chi-squared test is one.

M48

a) False: A Chi-squared test based on a 2×2 contingency table would be appropriate if the authors were comparing the percentage accepted at only two journals; as the authors are comparing the percentage accepted in three journals, they would need to use a Chi-squared test based on a 3×2 contingency table.

b) False: A continuity correction is required only when performing a Chi-squared test comparing two percentages; as the authors are performing a Chi-squared test comparing three percentages, there is no need to apply a continuity correction.

c) False: Although the number of papers accepted is relatively small, the expected frequencies in all six cells of the 3×2 contingency table are greater than 5. Thus, the Chi-squared test is appropriate in this situation.

d) False: The authors would need to combine the data from two of the three journals only if one or more of the expected numbers being accepted or not accepted in the three journals is less than 5 (i.e. if more than 20% of the six expected frequencies are less than 5). As the expected frequencies in all six cells of the 3×2 contingency table are greater than 5, there is no need to combine any rows or columns of the table.

e) **True**: As the authors are comparing acceptance rates (a binary outcome) in three journals, a Chi-squared test based on a 3x2 contingency table would be appropriate, noting that the expected frequencies in all six cells of the table are greater than 5.

M49

a) **False**: Neither factor has to be an ordinal categorical variable if the Chi-squared test is to be applied. Each may be ordinal or nominal categorical.

b) **False**: McNemar's test is used to compare frequencies when the data are paired (i.e. dependent), which is not the situation described. An exact test may be used when assessing the association between the two factors in an $r \times c$ contingency table in which more than 20% of the expected frequencies are less than five.

c) **False**: A continuity correction does not need to be applied to the Chi-squared test statistic if degrees of freedom are greater than 1 (i.e. if either factor comprises more than two categories).

d) **False**: The Chi-squared test statistic has degrees of freedom equal to $(r - 1)(c - 1)$ if the contingency table has r rows and c columns.

e) **True**: The Chi-squared test statistic has degrees of freedom equal to the product of $r - 1$ and $c - 1$.

M50

a) **False**: Using the Pearson correlation coefficient does not infer anything about the distribution of either of the scores, so there is no suggestion that the distribution of each score was skewed. A hypothesis test for the Pearson correlation coefficient relies on the assumption that at least one of the two variables is Normally distributed. If the investigators had checked out the Normality assumption before testing the Pearson correlation coefficient, we would be able to assume that at least one of the scores is Normally distributed.

b) **False**: As the Pearson correlation coefficient is negative, there is a tendency for the level of psychological distress experienced by the women to *decrease* as perceived social support increases.

c) **False**: Although the P-value indicates that the correlation coefficient is highly significantly different from zero ($P < 0.0001$), the magnitude of the correlation coefficient is relatively small (-0.36), suggesting only a moderate association between the two variables. In fact, the square of the correlation coefficient is 0.13, implying that only 13% of the variation in one score is explained by its linear relationship with the other score (i.e. a substantial (87%) portion of the variation is unexplained or random).

d) **False**: Although the correlation coefficient is relatively small (-0.36), the small P-value (P < 0.0001) does indicate that this association is unlikely to be consistent with chance variation. Thus, there is some evidence of a linear association between the two scores, even if this association is quite weak.

e) **True**: As the Pearson correlation coefficient is negative, there is a tendency for the level of psychological distress experienced by the women to decrease as perceived social support increases

M51

a) **False**: $-1 \leq r \leq 1$.

b) **False**: If $r = 1$, there is a perfect linear relationship between x and y, with one variable increasing as the other variable increases, and all the points in the scatter diagram lying on a straight line.

c) **False**: If $r = 0$, there is no linear relationship between x and y. There could be a nonlinear relationship between them.

d) **True**: Interchanging x and y will not affect the value of r.

e) **False**: The absolute value of r tends to increase as the range of values of x and y increases.

M52

a) **True**: The x variable can be measured without error.

b) **False**: The values of y are Normally distributed in the population for each value of x.

c) **False**: There are no distributional assumptions about x.

d) **False**: For each value of x, there is a distribution of values of y in the population: this distribution is Normal.

e) **False**: For each value of x, the variability of the y values in the population is the same.

M53

a) **False**: As the estimated parameter associated with height in this study is positive, this indicates that there is a linear relationship between thoracic aortic length and height, with thoracic aortic length estimated to increase by 0.1 cm, on average, for each 1 cm increment in height.

b) **False**: The equation enables us to predict the thoracic aortic length for an individual of a given height; it cannot be used and does not make any sense to predict the height of an individual with a given thoracic aortic length.

c) **True**: This is calculated as $1.7 + (0.1 \times 123)$.

d) **False**: Each 1 m increment in height would be associated with an estimated increase in mean thoracic aortic length of 10 cm ($- 0.1 \times 100$).

e) **False**: By multiplying the height variable by 10, the resulting equation would provide the impact on mean thoracic aortic length of a 1 mm increment in height, a value that is arguably less rather than more clinically relevant than a 1 cm increment. To provide a more clinically relevant estimate, the investigators could have divided their height variable by 10, to give an estimate of the impact on mean thoracic aortic length of a 10 cm increment in height.

M54

a) **False**: Goodness of fit of the regression line may be assessed by evaluating the square of the Pearson correlation coefficient between the two variables: it represents the proportion of variability of y that can be explained by its linear relationship with x.

b) **False**: If a test of the hypothesis that the true intercept is zero is statistically significant ($P < 0.05$), this provides evidence that the intercept is significantly different from zero, but does not give any indication about the slope of the regression line. There is no linear relationship between the variables if the slope is zero.

c) **True**: We generally choose to centre the explanatory variable when the intercept of the model does not provide a predicted value of the dependent variable for a meaningful individual.

d) **False**: We generally choose to centre (not scale) the explanatory variable when the intercept of the model does not provide a predicted value of the dependent variable for a meaningful individual. We generally choose to scale the explanatory variable if the interpretation of the coefficient for that variable does not reflect a clinically meaningful change in the measurement.

e) False: An outlier is not always an influential point. An influential point will, if omitted, alter one or both of the parameter estimates.

M55

a) False: The intercept of the multiple regression model provides an estimate of the predicted peak nasal inspiratory flow for a *female* of zero height and zero age – this type of individual cannot reasonably be described as 'typical'!

b) False: The interpretation of the coefficient for gender is that the predicted peak nasal inspiratory flow increases, on average, by an estimated 33.0215 (l/min) as the gender variable increases by one unit. As females are coded 0 and males as 1 (i.e. the value for gender is *higher* for males than females), this implies that the predicted peak nasal inspiratory flow will be *higher* in males than females on average.

c) False: Although 173.34 l/min would be the value of peak nasal inspiratory flow predicted by the model for a female aged 55 years who was 1.63 m tall, we would be using the model to predict peak nasal inspiratory flow values outside of the range of data used to generate the model, as the study is based on a sample of individuals aged 13–27 years. Thus 173.34 l/min is likely to be an unreliable estimate of the predicted peak nasal inspiratory flow for a female aged 55 years.

d) **True**: By recategorising females as 1 and males as 0, the parameter estimate for gender in the model would now be −33.0215 (again, suggesting that males tend to have higher peak inspiratory flows than females). Note that the intercept would now refer to a *male* of zero height and zero age, and it would increase by 33.0215 to allow for the recategorisation. Other than the intercept and the parameter estimate for gender, the other parameters in the model would not change.

e) False: By recategorising females as 1 and males as 0, the parameter estimate for gender would be negative rather than positive, and it would provide an estimate of the impact on peak inspiratory flow of females relative to males. The intercept would now refer to a *male* of zero height and zero age, and it would be increased by 33.0215 to reflect the effect of the recategorisation.

M56

a) False: If the computer output contains an analysis of variance table, the F-test will be testing the null hypothesis that all the partial regression coefficients are equal.

b) False: A given partial regression coefficient represents the average change in the associated dependent variable for a unit change in the explanatory variable, after adjusting for all the other explanatory variables in the model.

c) False: We can perform a multivariable linear regression analysis only if the dependent variable is numerical. We would perform a multivariable logistic regression analysis if the outcome variable was binary.

d) **True**: One of the reasons for performing the multivariable linear regression analysis is to determine the extent to which one (or more) of the explanatory variables is (or are) linearly related to the dependent variable, after adjusting for the other covariates that may be related to it.

e) False: Collinearity is present if two or more of the explanatory variables are highly correlated.

M57

a) False: Although it appears as if being retired is significantly protective against driving while sleepy in the univariable analysis, after adjustment for potential confounders, the odds ratio increased to an estimated value of 0.9 (close to 1) with a 95% confidence interval that includes 1. This suggests that after adjustment for confounders, there is no evidence of an *independent* association between driving while sleepy and retirement.

b) **True**: Although it appears from univariable analyses that being retired is protective against driving while sleepy, it is more likely that this association can be explained by confounding with lifestyle factors and working conditions, as the estimated adjusted odds ratio is strongly attenuated towards 1 and the confidence interval for the adjusted odds ratio includes 1.

c) False: Although the estimated odds ratio moved towards one after adjustment, its value (0.9) remained less than 1, indicating a lower rather than higher risk of driving while sleepy in those who were retired compared to those who were not retired.

d) False: The estimated odds ratio moved towards one after adjustment; however, the odds ratio does not tell us anything about the odds of driving while sleepy in those who were retired, only the relative difference in the odds of driving whilst sleepy in the groups of individuals who were and were not retired.

e) False: The outcome variable that was used in the logistic regression was driving whilst sleepy with a binary outcome (yes/no). Ordinal (logistic) regression would have been used if the outcome variable had a few ranked categories. Multivariable linear regression would be useful only if the outcome was a numerical variable.

M58

a) False: In the logistic regression equation, the exponential of the coefficient attached to a particular explanatory variable represents the odds of the outcome of interest (e.g. disease) when the variable takes the value $(x + 1)$ relative to the odds of disease when the variable takes the value x, whilst adjusting for all the other explanatory variables in the model.

b) False: Logistic regression analysis can be performed only if the outcome variable is binary. The explanatory variables may be categorical or numerical.

c) **True**: The model Chi-square (also called the Chi-square for covariates) tests the null hypothesis that all the regression coefficients in the model are zero.

d) False: The deviance (also called the LRS or −2log likelihood) compares the likelihood of the model with k covariates to that of a saturated model. Essentially it provides a test of goodness of fit, with a significant result suggesting a poor fit. The model Chi-square tests the null hypothesis that all the coefficients are zero.

e) False: An assumption underlying the logistic regression analysis is that of linearity. Another assumption is that the residual variance corresponds to that expected under a Binomial model. The dependent variable is not Normally distributed.

M59

a) False: The pregnancy rate in the sample was 0.106 per person-year (=60/565).

b) False: The pregnancy rate in the sample was 0.106 per person-year, or, equivalently, 1.06 per 10 person-years.

c) False: One pregnancy occurred in this sample every 9.4 person-years (1/0.106).

d) **True**: One pregnancy occurred in this sample every 9.4 person-years (1/0.106).

e) False: Based on the estimated rate in the sample, if each woman had been followed for 3 years, 71.55 pregnancies would have occurred (=0.106 × 225 × 3).

M60

a) **True**: To investigate whether the legislation had a greater impact in Edmonton than Calgary, the authors should test for a statistical interaction between city and calendar year. A significant interaction term would indicate that the change in helmet use from 2000 to 2006 is different in the two cities.

b) False: The authors adjusted for companionship as they believed that cycling with other individuals who also wore a helmet would encourage riders to wear helmets themselves.

c) False: Although it appears that the true impact of the legislation on helmet wearing is lower in adults than in children, the authors have not performed a formal test to assess whether this difference is statistically significant. It is possible that the differences seen (relative rates of 1.29 in children but 1.14 in adults) could be due to chance variation as the confidence intervals are wide (and the upper limit of the confidence interval for adults (1.27) lies within the 95% confidence interval for the estimate among children (1.20, 1.39)).

d) False: By controlling for city, the authors have allowed the absolute rates of helmet use in 2000 (the reference year for the analysis) to vary by city. By also including a main effect for calendar year, they have assumed that the proportional increase in helmet use in the two cities is the same. To assess formally whether the impact of the legislation is different in the two cities, they should include an interaction term between city and calendar year in the model.

e) False: Although stratification is one means by which the authors could investigate whether the legislation appears to have a greater impact on helmet wearing in Edmonton than in Calgary, this would be a descriptive analysis only. Thus, to formally test for a difference, the authors should not stratify by city but should incorporate an interaction term between city and calendar year in their analysis.

M61

a) **True**: Since the transformation of the latest triglyceride level was the logarithm to base 2, for every doubling in the latest triglyceride level (i.e. a 1 $\log_2$ increment), an individual's rate of experiencing a myocardial infarction was increased by 35%.

b) False: As the latest triglyceride level is log-transformed before inclusion in the model, the parameter estimate relates to a 1 unit increase on the transformed scale (i.e. a 1 $\log_2$ increment, or a doubling). The statement 'For every 1 mmol/l increment in the latest triglyceride level, an individual's rate of experiencing a myocardial infarction was increased by 35%' would be appropriate if no transformation had been taken of the latest triglyceride level.

c) False: It is unknown in advance what the impact will be of taking a logarithmic transformation of a continuous covariate in the regression model; this will depend on the true shape of the association between the covariate and the outcome. By taking a logarithmic transformation, the authors will change the shape of the assumed association – as a result, the *P*-value is unlikely to be exactly the same (even if the conclusion regarding statistical significance remains unchanged).

d) False: The assumed association between the rate of myocardial infarction and the triglyceride level (mmol/l) in a Poisson model would be log-linear if there was a linear association between the log of the rate of myocardial infarction and the triglyceride level when measured in mmol/l. However, as the authors have taken a $\log_2$ transformation of their triglyceride measurements before entering them into the model, they have assumed that there is a linear association between the log of the rate of myocardial infarction and the *log* of the latest triglyceride level (i.e. this association is not log-linear).

e) False: The choice of base of the logarithmic transformation has no impact on the association between the covariate and the outcome; thus, the *P*-value will be unchanged if the base is 10 rather than 2. However, the parameter estimate will alter to reflect the fact that the reported parameter now relates to a 10-fold, rather than a twofold, increase in the latest triglyceride level.

M62

a) False: As there is a higher percentage of men in those receiving the new drug, and male gender is associated with an increased risk of CVD, adjustment for differences in gender is likely to lead to a reduction in the relative rate estimate (as at least some of the apparent increased risk is likely to reflect the fact that, by nature of their gender, the group receiving the new drug has a higher underlying risk of CVD).

b) **True**: As the median age is higher in the group receiving the new drug, and older age is associated with an increased risk of CVD, adjustment for differences in age is likely to lead to a reduction in the relative rate estimate.

c) False: As the percentage of individuals who are current cigarette smokers is similar in the two groups, cigarette smoking is unlikely to be a strong confounder in this analysis.

d) False: Although the unadjusted relative rate suggests that there might be an increased rate of CVD in those receiving the new drug, we do not know what the independent association is between the new drug and CVD after removing the effects of the potential confounders.

e) False: Although the relative rate dropped to 1.10 after adjustment for known confounders, it is possible that there may be other unknown or known confounders that may still have an impact. Thus, we cannot conclude that the 10% increased rate in those receiving the new drug can be attributed to the use of this new drug.

M63

a) False: It is inappropriate to perform a Poisson regression analysis when interest is focussed on determining the relationship between a binary outcome variable and a number of explanatory variables which may be numerical and/or categorical, and where all individuals are followed for the same length of time. Logistic regression analysis would be appropriate in these circumstances. Poisson regression is appropriate when it is of interest to relate one or more explanatory variables to the log of the expected rate of an event when the follow-up of the individuals varies but the rate is assumed constant over the study period.

b) **True**: The exponential of a particular partial Poisson regression coefficient is interpreted as a relative rate associated with a unit increase in the relevant variable, after adjustment for all other covariates in the model.

c) False: The effects of the different covariates in the Poisson regression model are multiplicative on the rate of disease (if disease is the outcome of interest).

d) False: Extra-Poisson variation occurs when the residual variance is greater (not less) than would be expected from a Poisson model.

e) False: Variables that change over time can be incorporated in a Poisson regression model by splitting the follow-up period into shorter intervals in such a way that the value of the variable for a particular individual does not change in any given interval.

M64

a) False: The method of least squares is used to estimate the regression coefficients only in univariable and multivariable linear regression analyses. Maximum likelihood estimation is usually used for the other generalised linear model (GLM) models.

b) False: The link function in a multivariable linear regression model with Normally distributed residuals is called the 'identity link'.

c) False: The likelihood is the probability of the data, given the model, not the other way around.

d) **True**: Maximum likelihood estimation of the coefficients of the GLM is an iterative process that maximises the likelihood.

e) False: The adequacy of fit of a univariable linear regression model is determined by evaluating the square of the correlation coefficient, representing the proportion of the variability of the outcome variable that can be explained by its relationship with the covariates in the model. Usually goodness of fit of a GLM is determined by calculating the likelihood ratio statistic, often referred to as '−2log likelihood'.

M65

a) False: It is necessary to create indicator or dummy variables for categorical variables with more than two categories only if the variable is nominal. If the variable is ordinal, then it is either treated as a numerical variable or dummy variables are created for it.

b) False: An interaction between explanatory variables in the model is also called 'effect modification'. Confounding occurs when an exposure variable is related to both the outcome of interest (e.g. disease) and to one (or more) of the other exposure variables.

c) False: Effect modification occurs in a statistical model when the relationship between one of the explanatory variables and the dependent variable is not the same for different levels of the other explanatory variable. Collinearity occurs when two or more of the explanatory variables are highly correlated.

d) False: Using automatic selection procedures to identify the optimal model by selecting only some of the explanatory variables to be included in the final model is probably most useful when the model is to be used for prediction. These automatic selection procedures suffer from a number of disadvantages and so are not recommended when interest is focussed on gaining insight into whether an explanatory variable influences an outcome or in estimating its effect on the outcome.

e) **True**: A model is over-fitted when it includes an excessive number of explanatory variables.

M66

a) False: Selection bias in a clinical trial arises when the patients included in the study are not representative of the population to which the results will be applied. Lack of randomisation is likely to lead to confounding bias.

b) False: Increasing the sample size is not likely to reduce bias in a study.

c) False: The ecological fallacy results in a bias which sometimes occurs when we believe mistakenly that an association we observe between variables at an aggregate level reflects the corresponding association in individuals.

d) **True**: A confounding variable is an exposure variable that is related to both the outcome of interest (e.g. disease) and one (or more) of the other exposure variables.

e) False: A confounding variable is an exposure variable that is related both to the outcome variable (e.g. disease) and one or more other exposure variables or risk factors. Failure to adjust for the confounding variable may lead to finding a spurious association between the risk factor and disease or to missing a real association between them.

M67

a) False: Levene's test is not used for assessing linearity. Levene's test is used to compare variances and may be used, for example, to test the constant variance assumption in an unpaired t-test or a one-way ANOVA.

b) **True**: The linearity assumption in a univariable linear regression analysis is satisfied if the scatter of the points in a plot of the residuals against the explanatory variable is random.

c) False: The linearity assumption in a univariable linear regression analysis is satisfied if the scatter of points in a plot of the residuals against the explanatory variable is random. It is also satisfied if the scatter of points approximates a straight line when the outcome variable is plotted against the explanatory variable.

d) False: A sensitivity analysis is used to investigate the robustness of a statistical analysis. To do this, we use a slightly different approach to the analysis (e.g. omitting data or using a different method of analysis that does not rely on the same assumptions) and measure the impact of any changes on our estimates and conclusions.

e) False: A data set should only be analysed in a number of different ways (all essentially investigating similar hypotheses) as part of a sensitivity analysis. If the sensitivity analyses are to be presented, they should be described as such and distinguished from the primary analyses.

M68

a) False: If the investigators reduce the power to 70%, they would have to decrease the numbers required for their trial.

b) False: If the investigators reduce alpha to 1%, they would have to increase the numbers required for their trial.

c) **True**: If the investigators increase the power of their trial to 90%, they would have to increase the numbers required for the trial.

d) False: If the investigators now believe that only 60% rather than 70% of individuals in the standard-of-care arm will experience the primary endpoint, the investigators will have to increase the numbers required for the trial.

e) False: Increasing the minimum clinically relevant treatment effect to 15% will mean that the investigators will require fewer patients for their trial.

M69

a) False: Altman's nomogram is useful for sample size determination. Fagan's nomogram is useful for determining post-test probabilities of disease using a Bayesian approach.

b) False: An internal pilot study uses data gathered in the pilot study as part of the main study database. This is appropriate provided all details of the internal pilot study are documented in the protocol. In addition, the revised sample size estimate using the pilot study data must not be less than the original estimate, and the same smallest effect of interest must be used for both calculations.

c) False: A power statement provides details of all the relevant quantities that were used in a sample size calculation, including the power, and thereby provides a justification of the proposed sample size rather than the statistical methods.

d) False: The optimal sample size of a study will have to be increased if the significance level of the proposed test is lowered from 0.05 to 0.01.

e) **True**: If it is decided that the power of the study should be raised from 80% to 90%, the sample size should be increased to accommodate this.

M70

a) **True**: The CONSORT Statement provides a useful set of guidelines for reporting the results of a randomised controlled trial.

b) False: The STROBE Statement provides a useful set of guidelines for reporting the results of an observational study, not a meta-analysis.

c) False: The QUORUM Statement provides a useful set of guidelines for reporting the results of a meta-analysis.

d) False: The EQUATOR network was initiated with the objective of providing resources and training for the reporting of health research, as well as assistance in the development, dissemination and implementation of reporting guidelines.

e) False: It is generally necessary to report in a publication which computer package was used to analyse the data in the study, irrespective of whether or not the data have been provided.

M71

a) False: To identify the proportion of those who really do have proteinuria who are correctly identified by the test, the authors would need to calculate the sensitivity of the test. The value of 0.85 in the text is the area under the receiver operating characteristic curve (AUROC) – this suggests that a randomly selected man with proteinuria will have an 85% probability of having a higher albumin–creatinine ratio (ACR) than a randomly selected man without proteinuria.

b) False: This suggests that a randomly selected woman with proteinuria will have a 78% probability of having a higher ACR than a randomly selected woman without proteinuria. To identify the proportion of those with a raised ACR on dipstick who truly have proteinuria, the authors should calculate the positive predictive value.

c) False: It is the likelihood ratio for a positive test result that is calculated as the sensitivity divided by (1 minus specificity).

d) False: Given two randomly selected women from the sample, one of whom does and one of whom does not have an ACR > 30 mg/g based on urinalysis, the dipstick analysis will correctly identify the woman with proteinuria on 78% of occasions.

e) **True**: Given two randomly selected women from the sample, one of whom does and one of whom does not have proteinuria based on urinalysis, the dipstick analysis will correctly identify the woman with proteinuria on 78% of occasions.

M72

a) False: The sensitivity of a diagnostic test is equal to the proportion of individuals with the disease who are correctly identified by the test.

b) False: The specificity of a diagnostic test is equal to the proportion of individuals without the disease who are correctly identified by the test.

c) **True**: The positive predictive value of a diagnostic test is the proportion of individuals with a positive test result who have the disease.

d) False: The positive predictive value of a diagnostic test is the proportion of individuals with a positive test result who have the disease. It is the sensitivity which is equal to the proportion with the disease who are correctly identified by the test.

e) False: The likelihood ratio for a positive test result is the chance that the patient has a positive test result if he or she has the disease divided by the chance that the patient has a positive test result if he or she does not have the disease.

M73

a) False: The kappa coefficient was calculated as the authors wished to assess the agreement between algorithms 1 and 2 for distinguishing between lymphogranuloma venereum (LGV) and non-LGV infections.

b) False: Kappa values are dependent on the number of categories, with values tending to be greater if there are fewer categories. Thus, if the authors had combined some of the non-LGV subcategories, resulting in fewer categories overall, the kappa value would probably have increased.

c) False: Although it is possible to perform a significance test that would test the null hypothesis that kappa = 0, this is not really pertinent in this case as it would simply assess whether any agreement was likely to be real or due to chance, rather than whether there is good agreement between the two algorithms. It would be preferable to conduct a significance test to assess whether kappa = 1 (i.e. perfect agreement) in this setting.

d) False: As kappa = 0.90, the Landis and Koch classification deems this as near-perfect agreement between the two algorithms.

e) **True**: The kappa coefficient was calculated as the authors wished to assess method agreement between the two algorithms.

M74

a) False: Cohen's kappa is used to measure agreement when the responses are categorical, but it is equal to chance-corrected proportional agreement and not to the proportion of pairs that agree.

b) False: We can calculate a weighted kappa value to measure agreement only when the data are measured on an ordinal categorical scale and there are more than two categories of response.

c) False: The intra-class correlation coefficient is an index of agreement which takes values from 0 to +1.

d) False: The Pearson correlation coefficient is an inappropriate measure of agreement when the responses are measured on a numerical scale. This is because it does not take into account the extent to which the best fitting line on the scatter diagram, when one member of each pair is plotted against the other, deviates from the 45° line of perfect agreement.

e) **True**: If the data are measured on a numerical scale and the difference between each pair of responses is determined and their distribution is approximately Normal, the limits of agreement in a Bland and Altman diagram indicate the range of values within which 95% of the differences are expected to lie.

M75

a) False: A randomised controlled trial often provides stronger evidence than a cohort study, but this is not always the case. Whether it does or not depends partly on the problem at hand and partly on the quality of the individual studies.

b) False: Published papers do not always provide all the relevant information (e.g. on diagnosis, prognosis or therapy) required for an evidence-based investigation. Other sources include books, conference proceedings, reports, editorials and the like.

c) False: Using evidence-based medicine implies that conscientious, explicit and judicious use has been made of the current evidence in making decisions about the care of individual patients. In some circumstances, the decision may be based on the results of a relevant randomised controlled trial, but this is not always the case.

d) **True**: The number needed to treat (or harm) expresses the effectiveness and safety of an intervention in a way that is clinically meaningful.

e) False: An evidence-based approach is not restricted to conventional therapeutic interventions: it can also be applied to alternative medicine.

M76

a) False: The data collected conform to a four-level nested structure (level 1: children; level 2: class; level 3: school and level 4: city).

b) False: The child is the level-1 unit for the analysis; the child's class is the level-2 unit.

c) **True**: The city in which the children live is the level-4 unit for the analysis.

d) False: The data collected conform to a four-level nested structure (level 1: children; level 2: class; level 3: school and level 4: city).

e) False: As the child's class is the level-2 unit for the analysis, and two children selected from the same class are likely to be more similar than two children randomly selected from different classes, it is important to take account of class in the analysis.

M77

a) False: When analysing the data, failure to take account of the lack of independence between the repeated observations in each patient usually results in under-estimation (not over-estimation) of the standard errors of the estimates of interest and, consequently, confidence intervals that are too narrow and P-values that are too small.

b) **True**: A simple appropriate way of analysing such data is to base the analysis for each patient on a single summary measure that captures important aspects of the data. We then compare the values of the summary measure in the two groups using a standard hypothesis test such as the Wilcoxon rank-sum test. Alternative, more complex methods could be used, such as a repeated-measures analysis of variance (ANOVA), generalised estimating equations or multi-level models.

c) False: It is inappropriate to compare the mean responses at each time point separately using an unpaired t-test because this approach ignores the repeated-measures nature of the data and, because of multiple testing, is likely to produce spuriously significant results.

d) False: It is inappropriate to perform a one-way ANOVA comparing the means in the two groups at each of the different time points because, as with the answer to (c), this approach ignores the repeated-measures nature of the data and, because of multiple testing, is likely to produce spuriously significant results. It should be noted that performing the one-way ANOVA to compare the means in two independent groups produces an identical P-value to that obtained by performing an unpaired t-test on the data in the two groups.

e) False: If a linear relationship between the response and time is appropriate, a simple sensible way of analysing the data is to fit a single linear regression line for each patient, and then compare the two groups of slopes using a two-sample test such as the Wilcoxon rank-sum test.

M78

a) **True**: If the clustering is ignored, spuriously significant results may be obtained.

b) False: A random effects model is appropriate for the analysis of clustered data if there is evidence of statistical heterogeneity between the clusters. It has nothing to do with randomisation.

c) False: If a random effects model were used to analyse the data, it would differ from the model which takes no account of the clustering because, although they both incorporate random error due to the variation between level-1 units, only the random effects model includes random error which is due to the variation between clusters.

d) False: Generalised estimation equations (GEE) are also known as population-averaged or marginal models. Random effects models are also known as, for example, hierarchical, multi-level, mixed, cluster-specific or panel models.

e) False: The intra-class correlation coefficient expresses the variation between the clusters (not the individual units) as a proportion of the total variation.

M79

a) False: The P-value for the test for heterogeneity was 0.40, which suggests that there is no evidence of heterogeneity between the studies included in the meta-analysis. Thus, the combined estimate of the odds ratio can be interpreted as a reasonable overall estimate of the association between statins and atrial fibrillation, provided there was no evidence of clinical heterogeneity between the studies.

b) **True**: As the 95% confidence interval for the overall odds ratio includes 1 (the value of the odds ratio expected under the null hypothesis), there is no evidence that statin treatment has a genuine effect on the odds of atrial fibrillation.

c) False: As there is no evidence of statistical heterogeneity, there is no need for the authors to perform a random effects meta-analysis.

d) False: Although the estimated overall odds ratio for atrial fibrillation in those receiving statins compared to those receiving control was 0.95, suggesting a small reduction in the odds of atrial fibrillation in this meta-analysis, the 95% confidence interval for the effect included 1, suggesting that this association was not statistically significant ($P > 0.05$). Thus, statins do not significantly reduce the odds of atrial fibrillation.

e) False: Although the authors presented a forest plot in their publication, the purpose of this was to display the estimated effect (with associated confidence interval) from each trial included in the meta-analysis and that of the overall estimate. Had they wished to investigate the possibility of publication bias using a diagram, they would have needed to present a funnel plot.

M80

a) False: A component of evidence-based medicine is a meta-analysis which focuses on the numerical results in a systematic review. Its main aim is to combine the results from several independent studies to produce, if appropriate, an estimate of the overall effect of interest.

b) False: The hypothesis test of homogeneity in a meta-analysis tests the null hypothesis that there is no statistical variation in the effects of interest between the included studies.

c) **True**: A random effects meta-analysis is often used instead of a fixed effects meta-analysis if there is evidence of statistical heterogeneity.

d) False: The index, I^2, used to quantify the impact of heterogeneity in a meta-analysis does not depend on the number of studies included in the meta-analysis.

e) False: Publication bias in a meta-analysis may be elicited by drawing a funnel plot and noting whether the shape of the points is skewed or asymmetrical. The forest plot is used to display the estimates of the effect of interest, with associated confidence intervals, from the different studies.

M81

a) False: Although there does not appear to be any linear association between the tar content of cigarettes smoked and the hazard of mortality, smoking cigarettes with a tar content of >22 mg was associated with a significantly increased hazard of mortality (hazard ratio: 1.44) compared to smoking cigarettes with a tar content of 15–21 mg ($P < 0.05$). This is demonstrated as the 95% confidence interval for the relative hazard does not include 1 (the value expected under the null hypothesis). Thus, we cannot conclude from these data that there is no association between the tar content of the cigarettes smoked and mortality from cancer of the trachea, bronchus or lung.

b) False: Men who smoked cigarettes with a tar content of > 22 mg had a significantly increased risk of mortality from cancer of the trachea, bronchus or lung compared to men who smoked cigarettes with a tar content of 15–21 mg. Although we can say that the hazard of mortality is greater in the highest tar content group compared to that in the lowest tar content group, we cannot say anything about the significance of this difference.

c) False: Eyeballing the estimated relative hazards, there does not appear to be a linear association between tar content and the hazard of mortality. Thus, inclusion of tar content as a continuous covariate in the analysis would not necessarily lead to a more useful estimate of the association between tar content and mortality.

d) False: The reference group for the analysis was men who smoked cigarettes with a tar content of 15–21 mg.

e) **True**: Had the authors changed the reference group for the analysis to men who smoked cigarettes with a tar content of >22 mg, the relative hazard estimate for those smoking cigarettes with a tar content of 15–21 mg would have been less than 1. This is because the numerator and denominator for the calculation of the relative hazard in the 15–21 mg group compared to the >22 mg group would be the inverse of that in the >22 mg group compared to the 15–21 mg group.

M82

a) False: What is of primary importance in a survival analysis is the time at which the individual reaches the endpoint of interest (e.g. death).

b) False: Survival times are right-censored when the patients are withdrawn from the study or died from causes other than that being investigated before the end of follow-up.

c) False: 'Informative censoring' means that a patient was censored for some reason that was related to his or her chance of developing the endpoint of interest (i.e. the two were not independent).

d) **True**: The relative hazard is assumed to be constant in a Cox proportional hazards model.

e) False: The log-rank test in a Kaplan–Meier survival analysis is a nonparametric test (i.e. making no distributional assumptions) that compares the survival experience in two or more groups.

M83

a) False: The Bayesian approach to inference reflects an individual's personal degree of belief in a hypothesis. It is the frequentist approach that emphasises the role of hypothesis testing and whether or not a result is statistically significant.

b) **True**: One of the disadvantages of a Bayesian analysis is the subjective nature of the prior so that its specification is often criticised as arbitrary.

c) False: Fagan's nomogram is a diagram which can be used to interpret a diagnostic test result using a Bayesian approach. Altman's nomogram is used for sample size estimation.

d) False: In the context of a diagnostic test, Bayes theorem uses the likelihood ratio to convert the pre-test probability that an individual has a disease into the post-test probability of the disease.

e) False: In the context of a diagnostic test, the likelihood of a positive test result describes the probability that the individual tests positive for the disease if he or she has the disease.

M84

a) **True**: Any estimate of model performance that is calculated using the same data set on which the model was based is likely to be over-optimistic. Thus, if possible, it is preferable to assess the performance of a score on a separate (ideally external) validation sample.

b) False: Although the P-value from the Hosmer–Lemeshow test was >0.05, demonstrating that there is no significant lack of calibration, it was only just above this threshold, its value being 0.06. Therefore, the authors would not be able to conclude that they have presented strong evidence that the model is well calibrated.

c) False: Although the authors have validated their model on a separate (external) sample, the patients included were simply consecutive admissions at the same intensive care unit (ICU). Thus, although they have provided some evidence that the model may predict well in an independent data set, this data set is likely to contain a very similar sample of patients to the original sample on which the model is based. Validation on a data set from a different ICU would provide stronger evidence of transportability.

d) False: Although cross-validation is preferable to internal validation, the model performance is still assessed using the sample on which the model was based. A true external validation would assess the performance of the model on an independent sample.

e) False: The AUROC for the validation sample was 0.712; had the model been no better than chance at identifying patients who are likely to die during ICU admission, the AUROC would have been equal to 0.5. Thus, there is evidence that the model is somewhat better than chance at identifying patients who are likely to die during ICU admission.

M85

a) False: A propensity score describes the probability that an individual falls into one particular category of an exposure variable. A prognostic score provides a graded measure of the likelihood that an individual will experience the event of interest (i.e. the event is the outcome and not an exposure).

b) False: A receiver operating characteristic curve is used to give an indication of the ability of the score to discriminate between those who do and do not experience the event of interest. We use the Hosmer–Lemeshow goodness of fit statistic to assess whether the prognostic score is correctly calibrated.

c) **True**: Bootstrapping is an internal validation procedure which can be used to estimate a prognostic score and assess its performance.

d) False: The Hosmer–Lemeshow goodness of fit statistic may be used to assess whether a prognostic score is correctly calibrated. The prognostic score itself provides a graded measure of the likelihood that an individual will experience the event of interest.

e) False: A regression model is sometimes but not always used to generate a prognostic score.

Model answers for structured questions

S1

a) – c) Table S1.2 provides a summary of the type of variable, summary measures, error checks and graphical measures that would be used to display each variable.

d) On the basis of this small sample of data, it appears as if information on study entry date, age and gender is reasonably complete. Information is missing on risk group, ethnicity and Body Mass Index (BMI) for approximately 5–10% of cases. For lipid measurements (total cholesterol (TC), high-density lipoprotein cholesterol (HDL-C) and triglycerides (TG)) and the receipt of lipid lowering drugs (LLDs), the proportion of cases with missing data is much higher. If the characteristics of those with missing data on these covariates differ in any way from those of the individuals with complete data, bias might be introduced. The investigators would be particularly concerned if the probability that the data were missing was in some way related to the outcome of interest (i.e. experiencing a myocardial infarction (MI)). Furthermore, if individuals with missing data are excluded from any analyses, study power will be lost. The investigators could consider imputing the missing data in some way (e.g. by using multiple imputation methods) before performing any analyses. Of note, the outcome of the study (whether or not the patient has an MI) is captured only as a date; in this format, it is difficult to distinguish individuals who did not experience an MI from those who did, but in whom the date is unknown or missing.

S2

a) The standard deviation (SD) is a measure of *spread* of a set of observations; if we determine the difference of each observation from its arithmetic mean, the standard deviation is approximately equal to the mean of these differences. Thus the standard deviation indicates how far the observations are, on average, from the mean. The standard error of the mean (SEM) is a measure of *precision*. It tells us how good an estimate the sample mean is as an estimate of the true population mean. It is useful to quote the SD if we are interested in assessing the distribution of a data set. It is more

Table S1.2 Summary of the type of variable, summary statistics, error checks and graphical measures that would be used to display each variable

Variable	Type of variable	Summary statistics	Error checks	Values to check	Graphical measures
ID	Discrete numerical	n/a	Identify any values outside range	None	None
Entry date	Date	Median (range)	Identify any values outside range (1/1/2000–31/12/2000)	None	Column chart
Sex	Binary	% male	Identify any non-allowable codes	Lowercase 'f' for ID = 29	None
Age	Continuous numerical	Check distribution: mean (SD) if Normally distributed, median (range) otherwise	Identify any ages outside range (30–65 years)	Age = 24 for ID = '24'	Histogram or box-and-whisker plot
Ethnic group	Nominal	% in each category	Identify any non-allowable codes	None	Bar chart or pie chart
Smoking	Ordinal	% in each category	Identify any non-allowable codes	None	Bar chart or pie chart
BMI	Continuous numerical	Check distribution; if follows Normal distribution, then mean (SD), otherwise median (IQR)	Identify any values outside of a range typical for this age group (e.g. 10–40 kg/m^2)	None	Histogram or box-and-whisker plot
TC	Continuous numerical	As above	As above	Value of 111.1 for ID = 24	Histogram or box-and-whisker plot
HDL-C	Continuous numerical	As above	As above	None	Histogram or box-and-whisker plot
TG	Continuous numerical	As above	As above	Value of 13.3 for ID = 24	Histogram or box-and-whisker plot
LLD	Binary	% receiving LLD	Identify any non-allowable codes	Value of '?' for ID = 10; value of 'y*' for ID = 17	None
Date of first MI	Date	n/a	Identify any dates that pre-date study entry	None	Possibly Kaplan–Meier plot showing time to first MI during study

useful to quote the SEM if interest is focussed on the mean of the distribution, for example when comparing the means in two groups.

b) $SEM = SD/\sqrt{n}$. Thus the decline in forced expiratory volume (FEV_1) for the hospital and home administration data has $SEM = 8.4/\sqrt{602} = 0.342$ and $7.6/\sqrt{232} = 0.499$ percentage points, respectively.

c) The 95% confidence interval for the mean decline in FEV_1 (expressed in percentage points) is approximately equal to the mean $\pm 1.96 \times SEM$. For hospital administration, this is $-3.3 \pm (1.96 \times 0.342) = (-3.97$ to $-2.62)$, and it is $-3.5 \pm (1.96 \times 0.499) = (-4.48$ to $-2.52)$ for home administration of antibiotics.

d) The 95% confidence interval for the mean decline in FEV_1 for hospital administration of antibiotics may be roughly interpreted to infer that we are 95% certain that the true mean decline in percentage points over the period will lie somewhere from -3.97 to -2.62. More correctly, if we were to repeat the study many times, this range of values would contain the true mean decline in percentage points on 95% of occasions.

e) The median is a better summary measure of location that the mean when the data are skewed. Interval data of this kind are often skewed to the right and so, in these circumstances, the median interval would be a better representation of central tendency than the mean which would be unduly influenced by the few extreme (large) values.

f) The interquartile range is the difference between the first and third quartiles of the data. An interquartile range for the interval between courses of antibiotics for home administration of 155 days implies that the range of values of the central 50% of the ordered observations was 155 days.

S3

a) There was a moderate positive correlation between length of stay and age ($r_s = 0.4$), indicating that those who are older tend to have longer stays than those who are younger. This correlation coefficient was statistically significant ($P < 0.01$), suggesting that the association was unlikely to be a chance finding. The correlation between length of stay and MMA was somewhat weaker at 0.28, although it was statistically significant ($P < 0.05$), suggesting that those with higher MMA values were likely to experience longer stays in hospital. The negative correlation between length of stay and albumin ($r_s = -0.35$) suggests that lower values of albumin are associated with longer durations of stay. Again, the correlation was moderate but was statistically significant ($P < 0.05$).

The Spearman correlation coefficient is generally calculated (rather than the Pearson correlation coefficient) when the authors wish to describe the association between two numerical variables where one or more of the following applies: (i) at least one of the variables is measured on an ordinal scale, (ii) neither variable is Normally distributed, (iii) the sample size is small or (iv) the association between the two variables is believed to be nonlinear. In this situation, neither (i) nor (iii) applies. Therefore, we would assume that the authors have calculated Spearman correlation coefficients as they believe that many of the variables do not follow a Normal distribution, or because they believe the associations between them are nonlinear. Using the data in Table S3.1, we can calculate the mean $\pm 2 \times SD$ for each of the numerical variables, and this would provide the central range of most of the values if the variable is approximately Normally distributed. For length of stay, this range encompasses negative values, suggesting that this variable is skewed to the right (as negative lengths of stay are not possible). Similarly, the range for MMA also encompasses negative values (not possible for a measurement of MMA), suggesting that this variable has a right-skewed distribution. The ranges for age and albumin, however, do not indicate that these variables are not Normally distributed. It may therefore be possible to calculate Pearson correlation coefficients when assessing associations with these variables.

b) The authors have not presented exact P-values but have given a range of values within which the P-value lies (e.g. $P < 0.05$ and $P < 0.01$). Presentation of exact P-values is preferable as the information provided about the degree of confidence in the results is greater.

c) It is likely that the authors chose to present medians for plasma vitamin B6, serum vitamin B12 and plasma MMA as they did not believe that these variables followed a Normal distribution. For variables that do not follow a Normal distribution, the median is generally preferred to the mean as a summary measure to reflect the 'average' value. Where this is the case, the standard deviation is an inappropriate summary measure of the 'spread' of the values as the standard deviation incorporates the mean into its determination. Thus, it would have been preferable for the authors to present the range or interquartile range of values as a measure of spread rather than the SD for those variables not following a Normal distribution. As noted in the response to (b), it is unlikely that length of stay follows a Normal distribution – presentation of the mean length of stay is therefore not recommended. Further information about the shape of the distributions of the other numerical variables would allow us to assess whether the mean is an appropriate summary measure for each of them.

d) As the comparison is between two independent groups of patients, the authors would use either an unpaired t-test to compare the means (if the variable, or some transformation of it, follows a Normal distribution and the variances in the two groups are equal) or a Wilcoxon rank-sum test or Mann-Whitney U-test to compare the distributions (if the variable does not follow a Normal distribution).

e) A Fisher's exact test would usually be used to compare the proportion of individuals with a feature (in this case, >2 vitamin deficiencies) in two independent groups, where the expected number of patients in one or more cells of the table is less than 5. To calculate the expected frequency in each cell of the table, we multiply the marginal totals for that cell by each other and divide this product by the overall total. Using this approach, the expected number of patients in each of the four cells of the table would be 22.9 (<21 days, <2 deficiencies), 12.1 (>21 days, <2 deficiencies), 11.1 (<21 days, >2 deficiencies) and 5.9 (>21 days, >2 deficiencies). As all of these expected frequencies are greater than 5, the authors could have used the continuity-corrected Chi-squared test for a 2×2 table to compare the proportions with >2 deficiencies in the two groups.

S4

a) The design of a case–control study requires that a group of individuals with the outcome of interest (the cases) is compared to a group of individuals without the outcome of interest (the controls) in terms of their previous exposure to a factor. In this study, the outcome of interest is mortality and the factor of interest is age (over or under 65 years). Thus, if the authors had followed a case–control design, their cases would have been individuals who had died from their burn injuries, and their controls would have been individuals who had not died; the groups would then be compared to see whether cases included a greater proportion of the over-65 group than controls. However, in this study, the authors identified cases and controls on the basis of the exposure of interest rather than the outcome. As there was also some follow-up of patients (to establish whether they did or did not die), this study would more appropriately be described as a cohort study.

b) The mean and standard deviation (SD) are appropriate measures of location and spread if the variable is (approximately) Normally distributed. The median and range (or interquartile range) are appropriate summary measures if the distribution of the variable is skewed. The Normality of the distribution of the variable can be assessed by calculating the mean $\pm$ 2 SD; this range should encompass approximately 95% of values in the population if the variable follows a Normal distribution. Alternatively, if the data are Normally distributed, the distribution of the variable will be symmetrical with the mean and the median being equal, their value lying in the middle of the range of values.

The numerical variables in Table S4.1 are the percentage of the total body surface area (%TBSA), the deep burn surface area expressed as a percentage (%DTBSA), the proportion DTBSA:TBSA and the length of stay. It is clear that the median %TBSA is lower than would be expected if this variable was Normally distributed. This suggests that %TBSA is skewed to the right so that it is appropriate to summarise this variable by the median and range, as has been done in Table S4.1. The ranges calculated from the mean $\pm$ 2SD for %DBTSA and length of stay encompass negative values, which are not possible values for these variables. Thus, it is clear that these two variables also have right-skewed distributions and their distributions should be summarised by medians and ranges or interquartile ranges. Length of stay has correctly been summarised by a median and range in Table S4.1. However, it would be more appropriate to quote the median and range rather than the mean and SD for %DBTSA. The authors quote only the mean value of DTBSA:TBSA and do not present a summary measure for the spread of values of DTBSA:TBSA, so we cannot reach any conclusions about the shape of its distribution and cannot assess whether the mean is an appropriate summary measure of location. Similarly for the number of surgeries required.

c) The unadjusted odds ratio for mortality is calculated as the odds of mortality in the over-65 group divided by the odds of mortality in the under-65 group. We can estimate (based on the percentages given in Table S4.1) that 32 of the over-65 group died (i.e. 0.48 × 66) and 34 did not die (i.e. 66 − 32), giving an odds of mortality in this group of 32/34 (= 0.9412); we can then estimate that 53 of the under-65 group died (0.24 × 220) and 167 did not die (220 − 53), with an odds of mortality in this group of 53/167 (= 0.3174). Thus the odds ratio would equal 0.9412 / 0.3174 = 3.0 (rounded to one decimal place).

d) It is clear from looking at Table S4.1 that there are substantial differences between the two groups (e.g. the over-65 group has a lower percentage of men and a smaller median % TBSA). Many of the factors that differ between the two groups are also likely to be associated with mortality (e.g. men generally have a higher mortality rate than women and mortality rates are higher in those with more severe burns, as reflected in a greater %TBSA, the need

for more surgery etc.). Because of this, the over-65 group actually has a better mortality risk profile than the under-65 group and this could confound any associations between age and mortality risk. For this reason, the authors chose to perform a multivariable logistic regression which allowed them to remove the effects of known confounding factors. The adjusted odds ratio of 12.02 suggests that the odds of dying in the over-65 group is 12.02 times greater than that in the under-65 group, after controlling for the other factors in the model. The P-value of <0.001 suggests that this association is unlikely to be a chance finding. The adjusted estimate is substantially greater than the unadjusted estimate of 3.0, reflecting the fact that, if the over-65 group had a similar risk profile to the younger group, the mortality rate would have been even higher than the observed value of 48%.

---

a) To perform a true intention-to-treat analysis of the primary outcome of the study, the authors would need to know the outcome (i.e. whether the children did or did not experience a treatment response with resolution of diarrhoea) of all children who were randomised in the study. Unfortunately, 55 of the children randomised to A and 40 of the children randomised to B either were lost to follow-up or died before they could be evaluated for the primary endpoint. Therefore, these children could not be included in the analysis of the primary endpoint. To be included in this analysis, some assumption must be made about their likely response to treatment had they been followed for a sufficient period of time to experience the endpoint. For example, the authors may wish to take a worst case scenario by assuming that *none* of these children would respond to treatment, or a best case scenario by assuming that *all* of the children would respond.

b) By taking a worst case scenario and thereby assuming that children who were lost to follow-up or who died prior to evaluation of the primary endpoint had not experienced the primary endpoint (i.e. their diarrhoea had not resolved), the odds of a response for those randomised to A would be 0.9756 (= 120 / (243 − 120)) and that for those randomised to B would be 0.8095 (= 102 / (228 − 102)). The odds ratio for a response in A compared to B would therefore equal 1.21 (=0.9756 / 0.8095). Note that for this analysis, all children should be analysed according to the arm to which they were randomised, regardless of whether they did or did not receive the medication they were assigned by randomisation. These results suggest that the odds of a response among children randomised to A is around 21% higher than that among children who were randomised to B.

c) For a per-protocol analysis, it is likely that the authors would include in their analyses only those children who received the drug that they were randomised to receive. For A, this means that the calculations would be based on the subset of 143 children who actually received treatment A, whereas for B, the calculations would be based on the subset of 186 children who actually received treatment B. Using these data, the odds ratio for A relative to B would be ((76 / 67) / (100 / 86)) = 0.98. Rather than indicating that children randomised to A are likely to have a better response than children randomised to B (as in the intention-to-treat analysis in (b)), these results suggest that response rates among children randomised to A and B are very similar. Thus, the conclusions of the study do change. This is likely to be due to a combination of two factors. Firstly, a greater proportion of children who were randomised to A either were lost to follow-up or died before being evaluated for the primary endpoint compared to those randomised to B. As this group was likely to be the group with the poorer outcomes, their exclusion would have introduced bias. Furthermore, among those who were evaluated for the primary endpoint, a much greater proportion of those randomised to A switched treatments compared to those randomised to B. As switching treatments appears to be associated with better outcomes, this also may have introduced bias. Thus, the per-protocol analysis has given misleading results.

d) Of the 682 children who were eligible to participate, 126 declined to participate and a further 85 died prior to randomisation. Thus, only around two thirds of eligible children could be recruited and randomised in this trial. The results may not be generalisable to those children who are the most severely ill when they are assessed for eligibility (who are likely to be at highest risk of mortality over the short term). Furthermore, if there are any differences in the characteristics of children in the trial and those who declined to participate, then the results would be generalisable only to those children with similar characteristics to those in the trial.

S6

a) A power of 80% in the context of this study means that the investigators had an 80% chance of correctly detecting, as statistically significant at the 5% level, a difference of at least 10% between the two treatments in the recovery of continence.

b) The Type II error rate is 100 minus the power of the study (i.e. it is 20%).

c) The maximum chance of making a Type I error is equal to the significance level (i.e. it was 5%).

d) The power of the study would have been greater than 80% if the clinically relevant difference was increased to 15%.

e) The power of the study would be less than 80% if the significance level was more stringent (i.e. if it was 1% instead of 5%).

f) Although the investigators determined that they would need to randomise 96 men to each arm, they analysed the data when they had only 33 men in each arm. The study was therefore substantially underpowered, and it is not surprising that they did not obtain a statistically significant result. The authors should have provided an estimate of the treatment effect and its 95% confidence interval to add further support to their conclusions.

S7

a) The investigators used a paired t-test. The Wilcoxon signed-ranks test might have been used instead. It would have been more appropriate to use the Wilcoxon signed-ranks test because the differences in vitreal glutamate concentration between the left and right eyes are not Normally distributed. If the differences were Normally distributed, then the mean difference would be approximately equal to the median difference. However, these values are −0.6744 μmol/L and −0.100 μmol/L, respectively, suggesting a left-skewed distribution of differences.

b) The null hypothesis for the paired t-test is H_0: the mean difference between the left (with glaucoma) and right eye (without glaucoma) of the same rhesus monkey in vitreal glutamate concentration is zero in the population.

c) The main assumption underlying the paired t-test is that the mean of the difference between the left and right eyes within the same monkey is Normally distributed. It is also assumed that the sample size is reasonably large.

d) The mean difference between the left and right eyes is −0.6744 μmol/L, which is smaller than the median difference of −0.1000 μmol/L, suggesting that these differences are not Normally distributed (i.e. they are probably skewed to the left)

e) A two-tailed paired t-test is one in which the alternative hypothesis does not indicate the direction of the mean difference: the alternative hypothesis simply states that the mean of the differences is not equal to zero. This implies that the mean of the differences could be greater or less than zero if the null hypothesis is not true.

f) $P = 0.541$. This means there is a 54% chance of getting the observed results (i.e. a mean difference −0.6744 μmol/L), or one that is more extreme, if the null hypothesis is true.

g) There is no evidence to reject the null hypothesis, i.e. vitreal glutamate concentrations are not significantly different in eyes with and without glaucoma.

h) The 95% confidence interval implies that we are 95% certain that the true mean difference in vitreal glutamate concentration between eyes with and without glaucoma lies from −3.112 to 1.7623 μmol/L (when the concentration of the eye with glaucoma is subtracted from that of the eye without glaucoma). Strictly, on repeated sampling, this range of values would include the true value of the mean difference on 95% of occasions.

i) This confidence interval contains zero, which would be the value expected under the null hypothesis, implying that there is no evidence to reject the null hypothesis, $P > 0.05$.

S8

a) When performing a Chi-squared test, we make the assumption that at least 80% of the expected frequencies in the cells of the table are greater than or equal to 5. Although the authors do not report the absolute numbers in each cell of Table S8.1, these can be estimated using the percentages provided. With this information, we can then calculate the expected number in each cell of the table by multiplying the marginal totals for that cell by each other and dividing by the overall number in the study. These values are shown in Table S8.2. As all expected frequencies are greater than 5, the assumption underlying the Chi-squared test is met.

b) Using the data in Table S8.2, the Chi-squared value can be calculated as:

$$(12 - 5.9)^2/5.9 + (10 - 16.1)^2/16.1 + \ldots + (24 - 18.3)^2/18.3$$
$$= 6.3068 + 2.3112 + \ldots + 1.7754$$
$$= 15.2581$$

Table S8.2 Observed (expected) frequencies in each cell. Reproduced with permission of Wolters Kluwer Health.

Sense of coherence	Neuropathic pain	Non-neuropathic pain	Total
Low	12 (5.9)	10 (16.1)	22
Below middle	6 (6.1)	17 (16.9)	23
Above middle	9 (9.3)	26 (25.7)	35
High	1 (6.7)	24 (18.3)	25
Total	28	77	105

(Note that use of a computer package, which does not round the values, returns a more precise value of 15.332.)

This Chi-squared value follows a Chi-squared distribution with three degrees of freedom. Computer output provides a P-value of 0.002 for this comparison.

c) As the sense-of-coherence variable is an ordinal categorical variable, the authors could also have performed a Chi-squared test for trend – this would have provided a more powerful analysis as it would have taken account of the ordering of the sense-of-coherence variable. Alternatively, assuming that the authors do have the raw data for sense of coherence (and haven't simply collected the data in categorised form), the authors could have used the Wilcoxon rank-sum test to compare the distribution of values in the two groups.

d) If response rates are low, there is the potential for bias to be introduced. In particular, there would be concern that bias might be introduced if the individuals who failed to return a questionnaire at the 12-month time point differed in some way from the individuals who did return the questionnaire. In this study, the authors noted that responders tended to have higher general health scores than nonresponders. If individuals who experienced a decrease in general health over the study period were less likely to return their questionnaires than those who did not experience a decrease in general health, the finding of no change in median self-reported general health score might be misleading (as it would be based on a selected subgroup of the sample whose quality of life remained the same or improved), leading to attrition bias. As the magnitude of the bias is likely to be at least partly related to the proportion of individuals who failed to return their questionnaires, there is a need for the authors to minimise this number so as to reduce the potential bias.

e) As each individual has an assessment of general health at 3 and 12 months, the authors should consider the change in self-reported general health scores in an individual from 3 to 12 months as the variable of interest. They could then compare these 'changes' in the two groups using an independent samples test such as the Wilcoxon rank-sum test or the unpaired t-test. As the change in self-reported general health score is a numerical measurement, but is unlikely to be Normally distributed (given that the original measurement could take only integer values from 0 to 10), the Wilcoxon rank-sum or Mann-Whitney U-test would be most appropriate. This approach is preferable to comparing the median values of general health in the two groups at each of the two time points as this latter analysis ignores the dependencies in the data. If the change in self-reported general health score *was* approximately Normally distributed (possibly after some transformation), then as an alternative approach, the authors could use analysis of covariance (ANCOVA) or multiple regression to compare the scores at 12 months, using the 3-month value as a covariate.

S9

a) The mean (median) of the BIC rates (expressed as %) in the immediate loading and conventional loading groups are 70.3 (75.5) and 82.3 (84.5), respectively. Since the median BIC rate for the immediate loading group is greater than the mean, this indicates that the distribution is skewed to the left. The median BIC rate for the conventional loading group is slightly greater than the median, suggesting that this distribution may be skewed to the left.

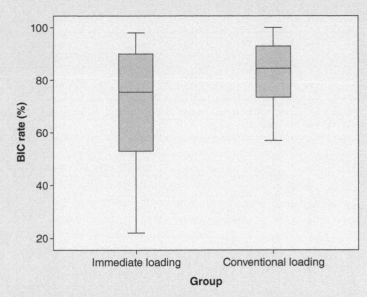

Figure S9.1 Box plot showing distributions of BIC% in the immediate loading and conventional loading groups.

b) Figure S9.1 is a box plot showing the distributions of the observations in the two groups. The distribution of BIC% is skewed to the left in each group. The median BIC% is greater in the conventional loading group, and the spread of the BIC% values is greater in the immediate loading group.

c) Since the data are not Normally distributed, the sample sizes are not large and the spread of the observations is not similar in the two groups, a nonparametric test such as the Wilcoxon rank-sum test (equivalent to the Mann–Whitney U-test) is preferred to the unpaired t-test. Its null hypothesis is that the immediate loading and conventional loading BIC% have the same distributions in the population.

d) This nonparametric test gives $P = 0.283$ (note: if performing the calculations by hand, the sum of the ranks of the immediate loading group = 98, and this value lies between 84 and 146 for samples sizes of 10 and 12 in Table A9(a) in *Medical Statistics at a Glance*, so $P > 0.05$). Hence, there is no evidence to reject the null hypothesis that the distributions of BIC rates are the same. However, it should be noted that the sample sizes are small and it may be that no significant difference was obtained due to low power.

e) Confounding bias may have been present because the palatal implants were not randomised to the immediate and conventional loading regimens. If factors likely to influence the histological bone-to-implant contact rates were not evenly distributed in the two groups, confounding bias could be present.

f) The estimated median (95% confidence interval), minimum and maximum values, 25th and 95th percentiles and interquartile range for BIC (all expressed as %) are shown in Table S9.1.

S10

a) The null hypothesis for the one-way analysis of variance (ANOVA) is that the mean shear bond strength (SBS) values in the population are equal for all the groups.

b) The one-way ANOVA assumes that the data are approximately Normally distributed in each group and that the variances are equal. A box plot of the data (Figure S10.1) indicates that the data are approximately Normally distributed in each group. However,

Table S9.1 Summary statistics for BIC, expressed as a percentage. Reproduced with permission of John Wiley & Sons.

	Median	95% confidence interval (CI) for median*	Minimum and maximum	25th and 75th percentiles+	Interquartile range†
Immediate loading	75.5	47 to 93	22, 98	51.5, 90.8	39.3
Conventional loading	84.5	72 to 95	57, 100	70.8, 94.0	23.2

*If determining the 95% CI for the median by hand using Table A10 in *Medical Statistics at a Glance*, then it is the second- and ninth-ranked values for $n = 10$ and the third- and 10th-ranked values for $n = 12$.
†The values of the 25th and 75th percentiles and of the interquartile range may vary according to the method used for their calculation.

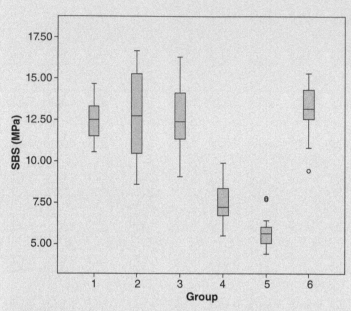

Figure S10.1 Box plot showing distribution of SBS values in the six groups.

Levene's test comparing the variances gives $P < 0.001$, suggesting that the variances are not all equal in the population. Thus, it would have been preferable to perform the Kruskal–Wallis test to compare the groups. This makes no distributional assumptions. It tests the null hypothesis that each group has the same distribution of SBS values in the population.

c) $P < 0.001$ in the ANOVA table implies that at least one group had a mean SBS value that was significantly different from that of another group.

d) It is customary to perform a *post-hoc* comparison test, such as the Scheffé test, to compare each pair of groups, as these *post-hoc* comparison methods adjust the P-value from each test to avoid a spuriously significant result arising from multiple testing. The more tests that are performed, the greater the chance of incorrectly concluding that the two means being compared differ.

e) The Scheffé tests showed that Coca-Cola (the positive control) and rosehip fruit tea had a significantly lower mean shear bond strength than all the other tea groups and distilled water (the negative control) (adjusted $P < 0.001$). There were no significant differences between rosehip fruit tea and Coca-Cola ($P = 0.215$), between any of the other tea groups (black, mint–maté herbal and mint–lemon herbal) or between these other tea groups and the negative control group ($P > 0.920$ for all these other tea group comparisons). It is of interest to note that all the adjusted P-values were very extreme (i.e. close to zero or close to one) apart from the comparison of Coca-Cola and distilled water for which

Table S11.1 Contingency table for association between 30-day outcome and endovascular repair (EVAR) versus open ruptured abdominal aortic aneurysm (rAAA) repair. Reproduced with permission of Elsevier.

	EVAR	Open rAAA	Total
Died	22	123	145
Alive	77	205	282
Total	99	328	427

$P = 0.215$. Since the adjustment for multiple testing has the effect of inflating the P-values, the conclusions would have been the same if unpaired t-tests had been performed with no adjustment for multiple testing.

f) It is reasonable to conclude that Coca-Cola and rosehip fruit tea may each be a causative factor in bracket–enamel bonding failure since they each had a significantly lower mean shear bond strength than all the other tea groups and the negative control group ($P < 0.001$).

S11

a) The contingency table of the results is shown in Table S11.1.

b) The 30-day mortality was $22/99 = 0.222$ (22.2%) and $123/328 = 0.375$ (37.5%) in the EVAR and open rAAA groups, respectively.

c) The Chi-squared test should be used to compare the 30-day mortality in the two groups. Its null hypothesis is that the proportion or percentage dying within 30 days is the same with EVAR and open rAAA in the population.

d) The assumption underlying this test is that the expected frequency in each of the four cells of the table is not less than five. This is satisfied since the four expected frequencies are 33.6 and 111.4 (for dying with EVAR and rAAA, respectively) and 65.4 and 216.6 (for being alive with EVAR and rAAA, respectively). Each is obtained by multiplying the relevant row marginal total by the relevant column marginal total and dividing by 427. For example, $33.6 = 145 \times 99 / 427$.

e) We find that the Chi-squared test statistic (including the continuity correction) is 7.25. It follows the Chi-squared distribution with one degree of freedom, $P = 0.007$.

f) There is evidence to reject the null hypothesis that the 30-day mortality is the same with EVAR and rAAA. The 30-day mortality is significantly lower with EVAR. However, it should be recognised that selection bias may have arisen because surgeon preference determined the treatment method in this observational study. Also, since randomisation was not used there may have been confounding factors that affected the conclusions, and no adjustment was made for these confounders in the simple Chi-squared analysis.

g) The additional information that should be provided is the difference in the 30-day mortality percentages with its confidence interval. The difference in the observed percentages is $37.5 - 22.2\% = 15.3\%$. The 95% confidence interval for the difference in percentages is 5.6% to 25.0%, that is:

$$15.3 \pm 1.96 \sqrt{\frac{22.2(77.8)}{99} + \frac{37.5(62.5)}{328}} = 15.3 \pm 9.72 = (5.6 \text{ to } 25.0)$$

S12

a) The authors wished to investigate whether there was a relationship between the proportion of doctors who agreed or strongly agreed with the statement and the year of the survey. As both variables are categorical, they would use a Chi-squared test to assess this. Since calendar year is an ordinal categorical variable, the authors can gain additional power for their analysis by using the Chi-squared test for trend.

To perform the Chi-squared test for trend, the authors would start by calculating the observed numbers who did (or did not) agree or strongly agree with the statement (Table S12.3.)

The Chi-squared test for trend (taking weights of 1, 2 and 3 for the three calendar years) would then be calculated as follows:

$$\frac{\left(\begin{array}{c}((1\times1111)+(2\times1382)+(3\times1195)) \\ -\left(3688\times\left(\frac{1\times3062}{7843}+\frac{3\times2036}{7843}\right)\right)\end{array}\right)^2}{\frac{3688}{7843}\times\left(1-\frac{3688}{7843}\right)\times\left(\begin{array}{c}(3062\times1^2)+(2745\times2^2)+(2036\times3^2) \\ -7843\times\left(\frac{1\times3062}{7843}+\frac{2\times2745}{7843}+\frac{3\times2036}{7843}\right)^2\end{array}\right)}$$

$$= \frac{((1111+2764+3585)-3688\times(0.3904+0.6999+0.7788))^2}{(0.4702\times0.52977\times(32366-7843\times1.86918^2))}$$

$$= \frac{(7460-6893.57)^2}{0.4702\times0.52977\times4963.78}$$

$$= \frac{320839.86}{1236.47}$$

$$= 259.48$$

This test statistic follows a Chi-squared distribution with one degree of freedom. Referring this test statistic to Appendix A3 in *Medical Statistics at a Glance* (or any other tables of the Chi-squared distribution) gives a *P*-value of <0.001.

b) Although female doctors were more likely to respond than male doctors, this would introduce bias into the assessment of time trends only if the relative proportion of female and male doctors has changed over time and if there is an association between the gender of the doctor and the doctor's likely response to the question. The authors could investigate this by testing formally (i.e. using a Chi-squared test) whether the proportion of female doctors has changed over time in the patients who have responded and by testing whether female doctors are more or less likely to agree or strongly agree with the statement. Furthermore, by using a multi-variable analysis (a logistic regression analysis would be appropriate) the authors could investigate whether any association between calendar period and the proportion responding positively to the statement is modified once gender is added as a covariate to the regression model.

c) To formally test whether any time trends differed between the two groups of medical school, the authors could have introduced an interaction term into a logistic regression model in which a positive response to the statement defines the outcome variable. The interaction term would be obtained by creating a dummy variable to identify the type of school (i.e. those that changed their course from 1999 to 2002 and those that changed their course from 2002 to 2004) and multiplying this by the calendar year variable (considered as a continuous covariate). A statistically significant interaction term would indicate that the time trends differ between the two groups of schools.

d) As the medical schools were not randomised to the calendar year in which they switched their curricula, there may be differences in the type of medical students attending the different schools and/or other differences in the education that is provided within schools that switched early and schools that switched later. These differences may introduce confounding if any of factors that differ are also associated with the individuals' perceptions of their readiness for work (e.g. some students may opt to attend a medical school that is thought to be ahead of its time in terms of rethinking the curriculum; this type of student may be more likely to feel that he or she is ready for work, regardless of the medical school attended). To alleviate any concerns, the authors would be advised to compare, if possible, the characteristics of students attending the medical schools that switched early with those that switched later. Similarly, the authors should attempt to compare any relevant factors in the didactic approach used by the two groups of medical schools.

S13

a) The intercept of the regression line is −29.14 kg. This would imply that when a child's mid-arm circumference (MAC) is zero, his or her weight is −29.14 kg, which does not make sense as a weight cannot be a negative number. This nonsense result arises because the regression line should not be used for values of MAC outside the range of values experienced by the children in the sample used to derive the regression line. No child can have a zero MAC, and so weight should not be inferred from the equation for a MAC of zero.

b) The slope of the estimated regression line is 2.94 kg per cm increase in MAC. This implies that as MAC increases by one cm, the weight of a child increases on average by 2.94 kg.

c) The 95% confidence interval for the Pearson correlation coefficient was 0.90 to 0.93. This is roughly interpreted to mean that the true correlation coefficient lies on or between these limits with 95% certainty (more exactly, if we were to repeat the procedure many times, the true correlation coefficient would lie between these limits on 95% of occasions).

Table S12.3 Observed number of doctors who did (or did not) agree or strongly agree to the statement. © 2007 Cave, *et al.*, licensee BioMed Central Ltd.

Year of survey	Agreed or strongly agreed	Did not agree or strongly agree
	Observed	Observed
2000/2001	1111	1951
2003	1382	1363
2005	1195	841

d) The slope of the regression line is significantly different from zero ($P < 0.05$). We know this because zero lies outside the limits for the 95% confidence interval for the correlation coefficient (i.e. it is 0.90 to 0.93) and so the correlation coefficient is significantly different from zero ($P < 0.05$). If the correlation coefficient is significantly different from zero, the slope of the line is also significantly different from zero (with the same P-value) because of the mathematical relationship between the correlation coefficient and the slope.

e) The regression line is a good fit to the data. This is apparent because the square of the correlation coefficient is $0.91 \times 0.91 = 0.83$. Thus, 83% of the variation in a child's weight is explained by its linear relationship with MAC and only the remaining 17% is unexplained (random) variation.

S14

a) A rule of thumb for multiple regression analysis is that there should be at least 10 times as many individuals in the sample as explanatory variables (covariates) in the model. There were 96 subjects with sleep apnoea, so it would not have been sensible to have more than nine covariates in the model. Six covariates is therefore an acceptable number of covariates.

b) The only significant coefficients were gender and upper airway length (UAL) ($P < 0.05$ for both). Thus we can conclude from the multiple regression model that upper airway length was a significant predictor of Respiratory Disturbance Index (RDI), after controlling for the effects of age, gender, BMI, HMP and soft palate length. In addition, gender was a significant predictor of RDI, after controlling for the effects of the other covariates in the model.

c) The estimated partial regression coefficient for UAL = 3.5 events per hour per mm. This implies that every mm increase in airway length conferred, on average, a 3.5-events-per-hour increase in the RDI, after adjusting for the other explanatory variables in the model.

d) The estimated partial regression coefficient for gender = −21.1 events per hour. Table S14.1 indicates that the reference category is 'males'. Thus the model shows that the mean RDI is 21.1 events per hour lower in females than in males, after adjusting for the other covariates in the model.

e) Providing confidence intervals for the partial regression coefficients is useful if the implications of the model are to be fully appreciated.

f) An R^2 of 0.6 suggests that 60% of the variability in RDI is accounted for by this model. However, this unadjusted R^2 does not take into account the number of explanatory variables in the model. The adjusted R^2 is more appropriate for multiple regression models.

g) The assumptions underlying the model are most easily checked by determining the residuals and the predicted values of RDI for each case. The assumptions are that there is a linear relationship between each covariate and the RDI (a random scatter of points should be observed when the residuals are plotted against each covariate), the residuals are Normally distributed with a mean of zero (a histogram of the residuals should follow a Normal distribution centred around zero), the residuals have the same variability for all fitted values (the scatter diagram of the residuals plotted against the predicted values should not exhibit a funnel or cone effect) and the results are independent

(this assumption is satisfied since there is only one set of results for each case). If the Normality and constant variance assumptions are in doubt, the P-values and the estimated standard errors of the coefficients may be affected. A violation of the linearity assumption is more serious: lack of linearity may negate the conclusions drawn from the model. Similarly lack of independence is important, and may lead to underestimation of the standard errors, confidence intervals that are too narrow and P-values that are too small, resulting in increased Type I error rates.

S15

a) The estimated odds ratio for age implies that the odds of progression to at least Stage III chronic kidney disease (CKD) increases by 5% for each one-year increment in age, after adjusting for the other covariates in the model.

b) The estimated odds ratio for gender implies that the odds of progression to at least Stage III CKD is 79% greater in females than it is in males, after adjusting for the other covariates in the model.

c) The estimated odds for preoperative eGFR implies that the odds of progression to at least Stage III CKD decreases by 5% for each one ml/min/$1.73\,m^2$ increment in preoperative eGFR, after adjusting for the other covariates in the equation.

d) Older age, female gender, greater tumour size, clamping of the renal artery and vein and lower preoperative eGFR were independently associated with newly acquired CKD Stage III or greater.

e) If we are not given the P-value for the odds ratio for any one of these factors, we can assess whether or not that factor has a significant effect on progression to at least Stage III CKD by determining whether or not the 95% confidence interval for the odds ratio contains one. If one is outside the confidence interval, the factor has a significant effect on progression to at least Stage III CKD ($P < 0.05$).

f) The use of logistic regression analysis in these circumstances can be criticised because the follow-up time in these patients is not constant. They are followed for between 3 and 18 months after surgery. An alternative way of analysing the data to assess the independent effect of these factors on progression to at least Stage III CKD is to use a Cox proportional hazards regression analysis or a Poisson regression analysis. In fact, the authors used both a Cox and a logistic regression analysis to analyse the data. They found that the Cox survival analysis produced the same significant predictors as the logistic regression analysis apart from clamping technique which was no longer statistically significant ($P > 0.05$).

S16

a) In unadjusted analyses, the first fracture (any) rate drops substantially from the lowest calcium quintile (17.2 per 1000 person-years) to the second quintile (14.7) – after this, the fracture risk remains relatively stable regardless of cumulative calcium intake (14.0, 14.1 and 14.0 for quintiles 3–5, respectively); a similar pattern in fracture rates is seen for the first hip fracture (4.6, 3.5, 3.1, 3.4 and 3.5 for quintiles 1–5, respectively). As fractures (and particularly hip fractures) are generally more common in older individuals, and the mean age at study entry is highest in the first quintile (it is 54.4 years in the first quintile and 53.8, 53.5, 53.3 and 53.6 years in the subsequent quintiles), we might expect the relative hazard for the first quintile (relative to the third) to be reduced after adjustment for age differences.

b) Unadjusted relative rates for the different quintiles are quintile 1: 1.23 (= 17.2/14.0); quintile 2: 1.05 (= 14.7/14.0); quintile 4: 1.01 (= 14.1/14.0) and quintile 5: 1.00 (= 14.0/14.0). These do not differ substantially (if at all) from the age-adjusted hazard ratios (HRs) reported in Table S16.1 (1.25, 1.06, 1.0, 1.00 and 1.00 for quintiles 1–5, respectively). In particular, despite the older average age of the women in quintile 1, the unadjusted (1.23) and age-adjusted (1.25) relative hazard estimates for quintile 1 are very similar. This is at odds with the conclusion to (a) that we might expect the hazard for the first quintile relative to that of the third to be reduced after adjustment for the different ages, although the similarity in the estimates may reflect the fact that the difference in mean age between quintiles 1 and 2 (<1 year) is very small.

c) The results suggest that first fracture (any) rates drop as the cumulative calcium intake increases from the first to the third quintile (i.e. the unadjusted relative rates are 1.23, 1.05 and 1.01, respectively), but beyond this level, fracture rates do not change greatly (1.01 and 1.00 for quintiles 4 and 5, respectively). This pattern is not consistent with a linear association between average cumulative calcium intake and fracture risk (for this to be the case, we would expect that the relative rate estimates for quintiles 4 and 5 would both be less than 1). A similar pattern is seen when considering the age-adjusted as well as the fully adjusted HR estimates for first fracture (any).

d) Unadjusted hip fracture relative rates for the different quintiles (relative to the third quintile) are quintile 1: 1.48 (= 4.6/3.1); quintile 2: 1.13 (= 3.5/3.1); quintile 4: 1.10 (= 3.4/3.1) and quintile 5: 1.13 (= 3.5/3.1). As for first (any) fractures, these are not substantially different from the age-adjusted HR estimates reported in Table S16.1 (1.51, 1.13, 1.07 and 1.12, respectively), and do not suggest a linear association with cumulative calcium intake (as the risk, if anything, appears to increase for the higher calcium quintiles).

e) A hazard ratio of 0.94 for any first fracture associated with a 300 mg higher calcium level implies that for each 300 mg increment in average cumulative calcium intake, the hazard of any first fracture is reduced by 6%. As the 95% confidence interval associated with this estimate (0.92, 0.96) does not include 1, a formal test of the hypothesis that there is no association between cumulative calcium intake and first fracture risk would return a P-value <0.05. Since the association between cumulative intake of calcium and fracture risk is assumed to be log-linear in the Cox regression model, the authors would need to calculate the logarithm of the HR (i.e. $\ln(0.94) = -0.06188$). They can then rescale this so that the

association reflects a 200 mg rather than a 300 mg increment (i.e. $-0.06188 \times 200/300 = -0.04125$) and then antilog -0.04125 to obtain the estimate (= 0.96). By following a same approach, the authors can also obtain rescaled estimates for the confidence limits (0.95, 0.97) as (0.97, 0.98).

S17

a) As shown in Table S17.2, fall rates are 10.6 (= 133/1253 × 100), 8.5 (= 12/141 × 100) and 5.9 (= 80/1366 × 100) per 100 rides for standard, Mark II and Mark III jump types, respectively, and 8.0 (= 150/1881 × 100), 6.7 (= 40/594 × 100) and 12.3 (= 35/285 × 100) per 100 rides for race distances of <3500 m, 3500–3999 m and >4000 m, respectively.

b) The unadjusted incidence rate ratios (IRRs) for Mark II jumps (compared to standard jumps) is calculated as 8.5/10.6 = 0.80. The remaining IRR values are calculated in a similar manner, as shown in Table S17.2.

c) On the basis of the unadjusted IRR estimates and their associated 95% confidence intervals (noting that a significant effect is obtained if the confidence interval excludes 1, $P < 0.05$) in Table S17.1, the authors would have identified that the fall rate decreases as the jump type increases, with races that involve Mark III jumps being associated with a significant reduction in the fall rate of 45% (IRR = 0.55, 95% CI 0.42 to 0.72) compared to races involving standard jumps. Whilst the IRR for Mark II jumps was not significantly less than 1 (IRR = 0.80, 95% CI 0.46 to 1.41), there is evidence of a trend to a lower fall rate for this type of race compared to races using standard jumps. The unadjusted IRRs for race distance appear to suggest that whilst there is no significant difference in fall rates between races of length <3500 and 3500–3999 m (IRR = 0.84, 95% CI 0.60 to 1.18), races of length >4000 m were associated with fall rates that were 54% higher than those seen in races of length <3500 m (IRR = 1.54, 95% CI 1.08 to 2.19). As the 95% confidence interval associated with this IRR estimate does not include 1, a formal test of significance would give a P-value that was <0.05.

d) Adjustment for the other factors in the model had only minimal impact on the IRR estimates for jump type, with the conclusions regarding jump type being unchanged (the adjusted IRRs were 0.74 instead of 0.80 for Mark II with a 95% confidence interval still including 1, and 0.51 instead of 0.55 for Mark III with a 95% confidence interval still excluding 1). After controlling for other factors in the model, the IRR for the association between a race distance of 3500–3999 m (compared to <3500 m) and the fall rate was reduced (from 0.84 to 0.76), although its 95% confidence

Table S17.2 Number of falls and rides, fall rate and IRRs for jump type and race distance. Reproduced with permission of Elsevier.

	Falls	Rides	Fall rate (/100 rides)	Calculation of IRR
Jump type				
Standard	133	1253	(133/1253) × 100 = 10.6	10.6/10.6 = 1.00
Mark II	12	141	(12/141) × 100 = 8.5	8.5/10.6 = 0.80
Mark III	80	1366	(80/1366) × 100 = 5.9	5.9/10.6 = 0.55
Race distance (m)				
<3500	150	1881	(150/1881) × 100 = 8.0	8.0/8.0 = 1.00
3500–3999	40	594	(40/594) × 100 = 6.7	6.7/8.0 = 0.84
>4000	35	285	(35/285) × 100 = 12.3	12.3/8.0 = 1.54

interval still excluded 1. However, the IRR for the association between a race distance of >4000 m and the fall rate dropped substantially from 1.54 (95% CI 1.08 to 2.19) to 1.17 (95% CI 0.87 to 1.58). The 95% confidence interval associated with the estimate now includes 1, so that a formal test of the hypothesis that the fall rate was not associated with the race distance would return a P-value > 0.05; this suggests that any association between race distance and fall rate is unlikely to be a real finding and the apparent association in the unadjusted analysis could be explained by confounding.

e) The authors believed that the association between the number of horses in a race and the fall rate might differ depending on the number of previous starts by the horse. For this reason, they combined the two variables in their regression model to provide exploratory data to give an indication of whether this was indeed the case. The adjusted IRR estimates appear to show that a greater number of starters in a race is generally associated with an increased fall rate, regardless of the number of previous starts of the horse. However, the IRR for >12 starters when the horse has had <5 previous starts (IRR = 4.51) is somewhat higher than if the horse had had 5–9 (3.19) or >10 (3.00) previous starts. We cannot tell from this model whether these values are significantly different (the 95% confidence intervals, which are 2.17 to 9.34, 1.69 to 6.02 and 1.62 to 5.53, respectively, exhibit considerable overlap so that it is possible that the association is the same, regardless of the number of previous starts). Thus, to formally test the hypothesis that the effect of field size on the fall rate is not related to the number of previous starts by the horse, the authors should include an interaction term between the two covariates in the regression model. A significant interaction would suggest that this hypothesis can be rejected.

S18

a) After adjusting for age, sex, genetic syndrome and surgery risk category, children of non-Hispanic white, other non-Hispanic and Hispanic ethnicities were 32%, 41% and 21% more likely, respectively, to die than their non-Hispanic white counterparts. The P-values reported in the table are all <0.05, suggesting that all three associations were statistically significant, and that the findings were unlikely to be due to chance. There is, therefore, strong evidence of racial differences in mortality rates.

b) Had the authors selected the Hispanic group as the reference group instead of the non-Hispanic white group, the RR estimate for the non-Hispanic white group would have been <1, reflecting the fact that the mortality rate in the Hispanic group is greater than that in the non-Hispanic white group. We can obtain an approximate estimate for this new RR by dividing 1.00 (the RR for the non-Hispanic white group) by 1.21 (the RR for the Hispanic group) to give 0.83. The RRs for the non-Hispanic black and other non-Hispanic groups would still be greater than 1, but would take values that are lower than their current values (non-Hispanic black: 1.32 / 1.21 = 1.09; other non-Hispanic: 1.41 / 1.21 = 1.17).

c) Had the differences in mortality rates between those of different ethnic or racial groups been fully explained by differences in access to care between the groups, the authors would have found that the RR estimates were all attenuated to one (i.e. no effect) after adjustment for the two additional variables. In fact, the RR estimates are not reduced greatly (and some increase), which does not support the

authors' hypothesis that these differences in mortality can be explained by differential access to care between the groups.

d) For the approach used in the fully adjusted model to be valid, the authors would have to assume that the two variables relating to access to care (insurance type and hospital of surgery) are perfect surrogate markers of access to care. If the markers were not perfect surrogates, then it is possible that there would be a residual association between ethnic group and mortality even after adjustment for the two variables. In practice, it is unlikely that insurance type and hospital of surgery would be perfect surrogates of access to care.

e) As some children underwent more than one episode of surgery, the entries in the data set could not be treated as independent. Had the authors not used a method that took account of the repeated measurements from some children, the standard errors of the estimates of interest would be underestimated, the confidence intervals would be too narrow and the P-values would be too small so that the results would be more likely to be significant.

S19

a) Errors in measurements may be random or systematic. A systematic error or bias is one in which the observed value tends to be above (or below) the true value. Random error or variation, usually due to unexplained sources, occurs when the observed values are evenly distributed above and below the true value. Thus, random error does not lead to biased conclusions and, in the context of this study, would not have been a contributory factor in identifying an association between birth weight and systolic blood pressure (SBP) later in life.

b) Publication bias occurs when there is a tendency to publish only those papers that report positive or topical results. In Huxley's study, although mention was made of the 58 published studies that did not report regression coefficients, the statistical analysis and the conclusions were based on the 55 studies which did report the regression coefficients. On this basis, it is reasonable to view the 58 studies without regression coefficients as 'unpublished' in relation to the analysis. Publication bias often arises when the results of small studies are not included in the analysis: small studies are less likely to produce significant results because of lack of power. The authors did, in fact, note a trend towards much weaker associations in the larger studies, consistent with the possibility that results from smaller studies were more likely to be reported only when extreme. There is a suggestion, therefore, that publication bias may have contributed to the findings. It should be noted in addition that, of the 58 studies that did not report regression coefficients and were not included in the overall assessment of the association, 23 of them did not observe a relationship between SBP and BW, whereas 52 of the 55 studies reporting regression coefficients reported lower SBP associated with higher BW. This lends credence to the possibility that publication bias was present.

c) Measurement error is usually defined as that which arises when a systematic error is introduced by an inaccurate measurement tool. However, random measurement error may also arise when the measurements fluctuate unpredictably around their true values, and it is caused by imprecise measurement tools, true biological variability or both. The bias introduced by random measurement error will be different depending on whether the error is in an exposure variable (BW) or outcome variable (SBP). Random measurement error in BW will bias the estimates of regression coefficients by underestimating them; this is called 'regression dilution' or 'attenuation bias'. In this study, most of BW values were obtained from birth records, but some involved parental recall or self-reports of BW (validated by comparison with birth records in samples), which may have involved greater errors. This may have led to regression dilution bias. By contrast, errors in the assessment of SBP would not be expected to produce any substantial underestimation of the association since, for a particular BW, any systematic error would simply add a fixed amount to the mean SBP and random error would not change the mean SBP, so the regression coefficient would not be affected.

d) Confounding occurs when we find a spurious association between a potential risk factor and a disease outcome or miss a real association between them because we have failed to adjust for any confounding variables. A confounding variable is an exposure variable (in this case, BW) that is related to both the outcome variable (in this case, SBP) and one or more of the exposure variables. It is possible that confounding was a problem in the 1999 study. The authors suggested that, amongst others, gender, parental blood pressure and parental socioeconomic status could be potential confounding factors. For example, socioeconomic status, linked to health-related behaviours such as diet and physical activity, may be correlated with BW and the SBP of offspring through intergenerational continuity of social conditions and health behaviours. Failure to adjust for socioeconomic status and/or the other potential confounding factors may have inflated the association between BW and later life SBP.

e) The authors of the 2002 paper were concerned about an inappropriate adjustment for current weight of the offspring. Some of the studies had treated current weight as a confounder and had adjusted for it in their analyses. Then those regression estimates would give an indication of the association between BW and subsequent SBP at a given current weight. BW is positively associated with weight later in life, and current weight is positively associated with current SBP. So, adjustment for current weight might produce a spurious inverse association even if BW and current SBP are uncorrelated. Current weight is an intermediate variable that lies on the causal pathway, and it should not be treated as a confounder.

S20

a) As each child was studied on multiple occasions, and the authors wished to incorporate the repeated measurements from each child into the analysis, they chose to perform a mixed-effects regression model analysis which took account of the hierarchical structure of the data set. Had the authors performed a simple regression analysis on the whole data set instead, the measurements in the data set would not have been independent, and this assumption underlying simple regression analysis would have been violated. As a consequence, the standard errors of the estimates of interest would be underestimated so that any resulting P-values would be too small, with results likely to be overly significant. In the mixed effects model, the annual visit for each child is considered as the level-1 unit, with the child being the level-2 unit.

b) From the univariable model, we can see that each additional hour of sleep that a child gets per day is associated with a reduction

in his or her BMI of 0.38 kg/m^2 on average. The 95% confidence interval associated with this estimate (-0.70 to -0.07 kg/m^2) does not include the value zero, suggesting that if a formal test of the significance of this association were to be performed, the resulting P-value would be <0.05 (i.e. a statistically significant association).

c) Adjusting for age and sex has very little impact on the estimate of the sleep coefficient from the model, which changes from -0.38 to -0.37 kg/m^2 after adjustment; this suggests that neither age nor sex are acting as strong confounders (although, since the relevant confidence interval for age excludes zero, older age is significantly associated with greater BMI). After further adjustment for maternal education, maternal BMI, income, ethnicity, birth weight and the mother's smoking status during pregnancy, however, the effect of sleep is reduced substantially to -0.24 kg/m^2. Furthermore, after adjustment for all these covariates, the 95% confidence interval associated with the estimate for sleep (i.e. -0.55 to 0.10 kg/m^2) includes the value zero, suggesting that the estimate is no longer significantly different from zero (i.e. we cannot rule out the possibility that the residual association with BMI is a chance finding). The only other covariates that have coefficients whose confidence intervals exclude zero are Maori ethnicity and a mother's smoking status during pregnancy. Hence these are the two factors that are most strongly associated with a child's BMI and it is likely that these are the two factors that most confound the apparent association between sleep duration and BMI. Further adjustment for lifestyle factors (i.e. physical activity, TV viewing and consumption of various food items) does not reduce the adjusted estimate further (it is -0.25 instead of -0.24 kg/m^2), suggesting that none of these factors is strongly confounded with sleep duration.

d) The adjusted estimate of -0.25 kg/m^2 in the full multivariable model suggests that a child's BMI is reduced by 0.25 kg/m^2, on average, for each additional hour of sleep that he or she gets in a day. However, as the 95% confidence interval (-0.56 to 0.06 kg/m^2) includes zero, implying that $P > 0.05$, we cannot rule out the possibility that this is a chance finding, and thus there is no strong evidence that there is a real association between sleep duration and a child's BMI.

e) The confidence intervals for the coefficients in Model 3 for age, Maori ethnicity, and a mother's smoking status during pregnancy all exclude zero, whereas all the other confidence intervals include zero. This indicates that these three covariates are the only factors that appear to have a strong and significant influence on a child's BMI in this study.

S21

a) Fisher's exact test is used on frequency data when the assumption underlying the Chi-squared test is not satisfied. The assumption is that the expected frequency in each cell of the contingency table is at least five. The expected frequency in any one cell is the frequency that would be expected if the null hypothesis were true and there was no difference between the proportions in the population of veterans requiring sedation receiving the water method and those receiving the air method. The expected value in a cell is the product of the relevant marginal frequencies divided by the overall frequency. They are shown in the column headed 'Expected' after the observed frequencies ('Observed') in the contingency table (Table S21.1).

Table S21.1 Contingency table showing observed and expected frequencies of veterans requiring sedation and veterans requiring no sedation in the air and water groups

	Air group		Water group		Total
	Observed	Expected	Observed	Expected	
Required sedation	27	33	39	33	66
No sedation	33	22	11	22	44
Total	50		50		100

All of the expected frequencies are greater than 5. Hence it was not necessary to perform Fisher's exact test. An appropriate test would be the Chi-squared test incorporating Yates' correction. This gives Chi-squared = 11.04, degrees of freedom = 1, $P < 0.001$.

b) The authors would have performed the two-sample/unpaired/independent samples t-test to compare the mean maximum patient discomfort in the water and air groups because the two groups are independent. This gives $t = 7.00$, degrees of freedom = 98, $P < 0.001$. The difference in means is estimated as 2.6 (95% CI 1.86 to 3.34).

c) The assumptions underlying the unpaired t-test are that the distribution of the variable in each group in the population is approximately Normal and the variances in the two groups are equal.

d) When the samples are large, the unpaired t-test is fairly robust to departures from Normality. However, it is less robust to unequal variances. If there is concern about the assumptions, then the P-value and power of the test may be affected.

e) In the water method group, the estimated mean maximum patient discomfort score is 2.3 and the standard deviation is 1.7. If these data were Normally distributed, approximately 95% of the scores would be contained in the interval defined by the mean $\pm 1.96 \times$ SD. However, $1.96 \times 1.7 = 3.3$ and $2.3 - 3.3 = -1.0$. Since the discomfort score is measured on a scale of 0 to 10, it can never be negative. Thus the distribution of maximum scores for this group is not Normal but is skewed to the right. In such circumstances, the mean is not a sensible summary measure of location, nor is the standard deviation (which is based on the mean) a sensible measure of spread. So, although the standard deviations in the two groups appear quite similar, suggesting that the equal variance assumption is not violated, neither the mean nor the standard deviation should have been used for these data.

f) If all the data are available, the Normality assumption in each group can be tested by eyeballing a box plot, dot plot or histogram and assessing whether the distribution appears symmetrical. Alternatively, the Kolmogorov–Smirnov test or the Shapiro–Wilk test could be used for a more objective assessment. The equal variance assumption can be assessed by performing an F-test on the ratio of the variances or Bartlett's test (recognising that these tests are not robust to non-Normality of the data) or Levene's test.

g) An alternative test to compare the maximum patient discomfort scores in the two groups is the Wilcoxon rank-sum test (equivalent to the Mann–Whitney U-test). This is a nonparametric test which is preferred when the data are ordinal: it does not make any distributional assumptions.

S22

a) If the hours for recovery are approximately Normally distributed, the unpaired t-test should be used to compare the average time for recovery in the two treatment groups. This test also assumes that the variance of the hours for recovery is approximately Normally distributed in each group.

b) The standardised difference for the unpaired t-test is the mean difference divided by the common standard deviation (i.e. it is $4/6 = 0.666$). Using Altman's nomogram, the line connecting a standardised difference of 0.666 to the power of 0.80 cuts the 5% significance level axis at about 70. This suggests that there should be approximately 70 patients in total, or 35 patients in each treatment group. (A more precise analysis, using a sample size estimation formula, suggests that there should be 37 patients in each group.)

c) If the power is 90% instead of 80%, the Altman nomogram indicates that the total sample size should be about 95, so there should be approximately 48 patients in each treatment group. (A more precise analysis suggests that there should be 49 patients in each group.)

d) If the investigators wish to detect a difference in mean recovery time of 3 hours, with SD = 6 hours, the standardised difference = 3/6 = 0.5. If the power = 80% and the significance level = 5%, Altman's nomogram indicates that the total sample size should be about 120 (i.e. about 60 patients in each group). (A more precise analysis suggests that there should be 64 patients in each group.)

e) Assuming that a total of 120 patients are required with equal numbers in the two groups, if the investigators want the ratio of the sample sizes to be 2:1, the adjusted overall sample size = $120(1 + 2)^2 / (4 \times 2) = 135$. Thus there should be 45 patients in the prazosin and antivenom group and 90 patients in the prazosin-alone group.

f) The Chi-squared test should be used to compare the percentage of patients achieving complete resolution of the clinical syndrome at the end of 10 hours after administration of the study drug in the two treatment groups.

g) If the investigators used a two-tailed Chi-squared test with an 80% power at a 5% level of significance, they expected about 20% of the patients in the prazosin group to achieve complete resolution of the clinical syndrome after 10 hours and they were looking for at least a twofold improvement in the prazosin plus antivenom group, the mean percentage = $(20 + 40) / 2 = 30\%$. The standardised difference = $(40 - 20) / \sqrt{\{30(100 - 30)\}} = 0.44$. Altman's nomogram gives a total sample size of about 170, indicating that there should be about 85 patients in each group. (A more precise analysis, using a sample size estimation formula, suggests that there should be 91 patients in each group.)

h) The suggested sample size is 35 patients in each treatment group for (b) and 85 patients in each treatment group for (g). Since both variables are of primary importance, the larger number should be chosen for the sample size (i.e. there should be 85 patients in each treatment group). It should be noted that it would be prudent to have an even larger sample size because of multiple testing (i.e. two hypothesis tests are to be performed) and its effect on the P-values.

Table S23.1 Contingency table showing numbers of mild Alzheimer's patients and healthy controls with a TYM $\leq$ or > 42

	Alzheimer's disease	Healthy controls	Total
TYM ≤ 42 (+ve)	$a = 87$	$b = 39$	126
TYM > 42 (−ve)	$c = 70$	$d = 243$	250
Total	94	282	376

S23

a) The sensitivity of a diagnostic test is the proportion or percentage of individuals with the disease (i.e. mild Alzheimer's) who are correctly identified by the test. The specificity is the proportion or percentage of individuals without the disease (i.e. the controls) who are correctly identified by the test. A sensitivity of 92.5% suggests that the TYM ('test your memory') self-administered test is very good at identifying those with mild Alzheimer's disease. The specificity of 86.2% suggests that the test is good at identifying those without mild Alzheimer's disease.

b) A contingency table (Table S23.1) shows the numbers of mild Alzheimer's patients and healthy controls with a TYM ≤ 42 and > 42. The sensitivity $= 0.925 = a/94$, so $a = 0.925 \times 94 = 87$. The specificity $= 0.862 = d/28$, so $d = 0.862 \times 282 = 243$. Then, $c = 94 - 87 = 70$ and $b = 282 - 243 = 39$.

c) The PPV is the proportion of individuals with a positive test result (TYM ≤ 42) who have the disease (mild Alzheimer's) $= 87/126 = 0.690$ or 69.0%. The NPV is the proportion of individuals with a negative test result (TYM > 42) who do not have the disease (controls) $= 243/250 = 0.972$ or 97.2%. The NPV is very high so if an individual has a TYM > 42, he or she is very unlikely to have mild Alzheimer's disease. However, the PPV is only 69% so that if he or she has a TYM ≤ 42, there is a reasonable chance that he or she has mild Alzheimer's disease but it is not nearly as clear-cut as the NPV result.

d) The ROC curve is constructed by evaluating the sensitivity and specificity for different potential cut-offs of the TYM, and plotting the sensitivity (true positive result) against 100 minus the specificity (false positive result), when both are expressed as percentages. The area under the ROC curve represents the probability that a randomly chosen mild Alzheimer's disease individual has a higher predicted probability of having mild Alzheimer's disease than a randomly chosen individual from the control group. A test which is perfect at discriminating between the two disease outcomes has an area under the ROC curve of one. The area under the ROC curve for the TYM is 0.95, which is very close to the maximum value of one, indicating that the TYM is a very good test for discriminating between mild Alzheimer's disease and control individuals.

e) The prevalence of mild Alzheimer's disease in this group of individuals $= 94/376 = 0.25$ or 25%. The prevalence of mild Alzheimer's disease does not greatly affect the value of the sensitivity or specificity of the test. However, the PPV will decrease and the NPV will increase in value as the prevalence of Alzheimer's disease decreases in the population.

f) It is not appropriate to use the prevalence determined in (e) as an estimate of the prevalence of mild Alzheimer's disease in the population because the individuals in the study were not randomly selected from the population. The controls were specifically chosen so that there was a ratio of 1:3 of cases to controls (i.e. there were 94 subjects with Alzheimer's disease and the investigators deliberately chose three times as many matched controls).

g) Raising the cut-off of TYM would increase the sensitivity and decrease the specificity. Lowering the cut-off would decrease the sensitivity and increase the specificity.

h) The likelihood ratio of a positive test result = sensitivity / (100 − specificity) = 92.5 / (100 − 86.2) = 6.7. This indicates that a positive test result (TYM ≤ 42) is nearly seven times more likely to occur in an individual who has mild Alzheimer's disease than in a control individual.

S24

a) The area under the receiver operating characteristic curve (AUROC) gives an indication of the ability of the score to discriminate between individuals diagnosed with alcoholic hepatitis in Denmark from 1999 to 2008 who do and do not die in a particular study period. The AUROC is estimated by selecting all 'pairs' of individuals in the study, one of whom does die and one of whom does not, and by calculating the proportion of these pairs in whom the predicted score is higher in the individual who does die. Alternatively, the ROC curve can be plotted and the AUROC calculated by estimating the area under the curve. The AUROC for the Lille score of 0.78 for 28-day mortality suggests that given any two randomly chosen individuals with alcoholic hepatitis, one of whom does die and one of whom does not, the score is able to correctly discriminate between these two individuals on 78% of occasions.

b) Whilst, for 28-day mortality, the Lille score has the highest AUROC value (0.78), AUROC values for all five scores are reasonably high and differences between them are slight (the other AUROC values are 0.74, 0.74, 0.75 and 0.76). Thus, all five scores have similar discriminative ability for identifying individuals at high risk of death in the first 28 days after diagnosis of alcoholic hepatitis. As the period over which mortality is measured lengthens, the AUROC values for MELD, MELD-Na and GAHS generally drop (for each consecutive period they are 0.74, 0.70, 0.67 (MELD), 0.74, 0.69, 0.65 (MELD-Na) and 0.75, 0.72, 0.69 (GAHS)) suggesting that their ability to discriminate between those who will and those who will not die decreases over the longer term. The exceptions to this are the Lille score (the AUROC is 0.78, 0.77 and 0.75 for the three consecutive periods, showing very little change) and the ABIC score (the AUROC is 0.76, 0.76 and 0.72 for the three consecutive periods, dropping only after the 84-day period).

c) Sensitivity: the number of patients with a MELD score > 21 who died within the first 84 days divided by the total number of individuals who died within the first 84 days.
Specificity: the number of patients with a MELD score < 21 who did not die within the first 84 days divided by the total number of individuals who did not die within the first 84 days.
PPV: the number of patients with a MELD score > 21 who died within the first 84 days divided by the total number of individuals with a MELD score > 21.
NPV: the number of patients with a MELD score < 21 who did not die within the first 84 days divided by the total number of individuals with a MELD score < 21.

d) Overall, the highest sensitivities for 84-day mortality are obtained when using the ABIC (6.71 threshold), MELD-Na and ABIC scores (0.92, 0.81 and 0.76, respectively); the highest specificity is obtained when using the ABIC (9 threshold) score (specificity = 0.87) followed by the GAHS (0.72), MELD (0.70) and Lille (0.69) scores. PPV values are modest for all scores (ranging from 0.27 to 0.43), whereas NPV values are high for all (ranging from 0.83 to 0.94). The sensitivities of all of the scores generally drop as the period over which mortality is assessed lengthens, whereas the specificities remain relatively stable; the PPV values generally increase, whereas NPV values decrease. If the primary aim is to be able to identify as many of the individuals who are likely to die as possible, then the recommendation would be to use the ABIC score with a 6.71 threshold, as this produces the highest sensitivity at all time points; if, however, clinicians wish to ensure that they have correctly identified those patients who are likely to survive, the ABIC score with the threshold of 9 would be preferable, as this has the highest specificity at all time points. The low PPV values, however, emphasise the fact that for an individual patient, a high ABIC score does not necessarily translate into a high mortality risk, especially over the first 28 days.

e) The low PPV and high NPV values are likely to reflect the fact that the proportion of patients who died over the study period was relatively low within the first 28 days (16%) – as a result, PPV values will be low on the whole with NPV values being higher. As the period over which mortality is assessed lengthens, a higher proportion of patients die (27% at 84 days and 40% at 180 days) and thus the PPV values gradually increase and NPV values decrease.

S25

a) To calculate kappa, we start by summing the observed frequencies along the diagonal of Table S25.1 (O_d = 718 + 164 + 17 = 899), and then do the same for the expected frequencies (E_d = 587.34 + 63.98 + 1.13 = 652.45). Kappa is then calculated as follows:

$$((899/1112) - (652.45/1112))/(1 - (652.45/1112))$$
$$= (0.80845 - 0.58673)/(1 - 0.58673)$$
$$= 0.22172/0.41327$$
$$= 0.537$$

As kappa lies between 0.41 and 0.60, this demonstrates moderate agreement between the two scores. Since both of the scores are ordinal, we might determine a weighted kappa instead, which takes into account the extent to which the two scores disagree. The weighted kappa is 0.573 using a linear weighting.

b) The authors have demonstrated moderate agreement between the two scores. However, as they do not provide results from a gold-standard test for liver failure, they have not assessed the reliability of either score to identify those with liver failure. Had this been the primary aim of the study, the authors would have been advised to identify patients who were undergoing liver biopsy (which gives a more accurate assessment of liver failure) and thereby establish who did and who did not have liver failure. Within this subgroup of liver biopsy patients, they could then evaluate the sensitivity and specificity of each score to assess its reliability for identifying those with liver failure.

c) Kappa values are generally larger when the number of categories is smaller. Had the authors combined Classes 2 and 3 for the purposes of calculating kappa, the number of categories would have been reduced and the agreement would therefore almost certainly have been greater.

S26

a) A formal way of assessing the systematic effect is to perform a paired t-test. This test makes an assumption that the differences are Normally distributed. If the differences are Normally distributed, the mean $\pm$ 1.96 SD should show the spread of most of the observations. Since the mean of the differences is 0.01 hours and their standard deviation is 0.5 hours, 95% of the observations would be expected to lie between −0.97 and 0.99 hours. This appears to be a reasonable assumption if we eyeball the Bland and Altman diagram and consider the distribution of points in relation to the vertical axis representing the difference between the two assessments. The test statistic for the paired t-test is equal to the mean difference divided by its standard error. Therefore, the test statistic, ignoring its sign, is equal to 0.01 / (0.5 / $\sqrt{43}$) = 0.13. This follows a t-distribution on 43 − 1 = 42 degrees of freedom, giving P = 0.90. There is no evidence to reject the null hypothesis that the true mean difference is zero, indicating that there is no evidence of a systematic effect.

b) The limits of agreement are equal to the mean difference $\pm$ 1.96 times the standard deviation of the differences. Thus the limits of agreement are equal to 0.01 $\pm$ (1.96 $\times$ 0.5), namely −0.97 hours and 0.99 hours (i.e. the dotted lines in the Bland and Altman diagram). In a population of such patients, we would expect approximately 95% of the differences in hours walked between the two assessments to lie between these limits.

c) It is sensible to calculate a single measure of repeatability because there is no evidence of a funnel effect in the scatter of points in the Bland and Altman, nor do the points show any evidence of an upwards or downwards trend.

d) The British Standards Institution repeatability coefficient is equal to 1.96 times the standard deviation of the differences. It is therefore equal to 1.96 times 0.5 = 0.98 hours. It represents the maximum likely difference in the hours walked between the two assessments.

e) From the Bland and Altman diagram (Figure S26.1), there is a suggestion that the mean number of hours walked by a patient in 24 hours was between 1.0 and 1.5 hours. The maximum likely difference between the hours walked in the 2 assessments was 0.98 hours (i.e. the British Standards Institution repeatability coefficient). This is a large number when looked at in relation to the average hours walked. Hence, it can be inferred that 24-hour AM monitoring of hours walked in ambulatory patients with MS is not very repeatable.

f) If we plot the number of hours walked in one assessment against that in the second assessment in a scatter diagram, using the same scale of measurement on both axes, the Pearson correlation coefficient between the first and second assessments of hours walked assesses the closeness of the data to the line of best fit. It does not give any indication of how far the line of best fit is from the 45° line through the origin, the latter indicating perfect agreement. It is possible for the Pearson correlation coefficient to be equal to one when there is no agreement at all between the pairs of values.

g) The intra-class correlation coefficient, such as Lin's concordance correlation coefficient, is an index of reliability. It is equal to one when there is perfect agreement between the repeated observations.

a) The null hypothesis for a test investigating heterogeneity in a meta-analysis is that there is no difference between the true effects of interest (odds ratios) in the included studies (i.e. they are homogeneous). I^2 represents the proportion or percentage of the total variation across studies due to statistical heterogeneity. When expressed as a percentage, it takes a value from 0% to 100%, with a value of 0% indicating no observed heterogeneity.

b) When all 11 studies were analysed together, there was strong evidence of statistical heterogeneity (test for heterogeneity $\chi^2 = 25.94$, degrees of freedom = 10, $P = 0.004$). In addition, $I^2 = 61\%$, indicating that 61% of the total variation across the studies was due to statistical heterogeneity. These two results do not necessarily imply that the source of the heterogeneity was the quality of the study. However, since the authors had determined the odds ratio separately for each study, they were able to assess that the probable source of much of the heterogeneity was the quality of the study, as demonstrated in the forest plot (Figure S27.1). Therefore, they judged that it was appropriate to perform a separate meta-analysis for the high- and low-quality studies. It should be noted that an alternative approach which recognises the statistical heterogeneity between the studies is to perform a random effects meta-analysis on all 11 studies. The investigators performed such an analysis, finding a nonsignificant overall odds ratio of 0.79 (95% confidence interval 0.58 to 1.06, $P = 0.12$). However, because of statistical heterogeneity, in large part due to the quality of the studies, it is more sensible to perform subgroup analyses for the high- and low-quality studies, as was done.

c) A fixed-effect analysis was used for the high- and low-quality studies because, in each case, there was no evidence of statistical heterogeneity and I^2 was zero or almost non-existent. In the high-quality studies, $\chi^2 = 4.02$, df = 4, $P = 0.40$, $I^2 = 1\%$: in the low-quality studies, $\chi^2 = 4.95$, df = 5, $P = 0.42$, $I^2 = 0\%$.

d) The area of the each box, representing the estimated odds ratio in a study, is proportional to the number of individuals in the study. Studies with large sample sizes will have bigger boxes than those with small sample sizes.

e) The overall odds ratio for the high-quality studies was estimated as 1.15 (95% CI 0.95 to 1.40). This means that the odds of preterm birth <37 weeks of gestation was estimated to be 15% greater in those women who had treatment with scaling and planing for periodontal disease during pregnancy than in those women who had no treatment (although this association was not statistically significant). The high-quality studies result suggests that treatment with scaling and planning during pregnancy could increase the preterm birth rate! In contrast, the overall odds ratio for the low-quality studies was estimated as 0.52 (95% CI 0.38 to 0.72). This means that the odds of preterm birth <37 weeks of gestation was estimated to be 48% lower in those women who had treatment with scaling and planing for periodontal disease during pregnancy than in those women who had no treatment.

f) For the high-quality studies, the test for the overall effect indicated that the odds ratio was not significantly different from one ($z = 1.45$, $P = 0.15$). Thus, although the odds ratio suggested that treatment increased the preterm birth rate, this was not a statistically significant effect. Furthermore, given the larger number of participants included in the high-quality studies, this lack of association is unlikely to be due to low power. For the low-quality studies, the test for the overall effect indicated that the odds ratio was significantly less than one ($z = 4.01$, $P < 0.001$). Much greater emphasis should be placed on the results from the high-quality studies, noting, in particular, that these studies had large patient numbers. Thus we may conclude that treatment with scaling and root planing for periodontal disease in pregnancy does not appear to reduce the preterm birth rate.

g) The effect estimate on the horizontal axis of the funnel plot is likely to represent the logarithm of the estimated odds ratio.

h) The funnel plot is used to assess the presence of publication bias. The funnel plot was asymmetrical; less precise (smaller) studies reported inflated outcomes in favour of the treatment arm (i.e. were more strongly associated with a lower odds of pre-term delivery) than did larger studies. Trials perceived to be missing were in parts of the funnel plot where no statistical significance existed, suggesting the presence of publication bias. However, given that publication bias usually involves trials with 'negative' results, any unpublished trial would be highly unlikely to have favoured the treatment arm. Thus, in spite of there being evidence of publication bias, the overall conclusion (that there is no evidence that scaling and planing to treat periodontal disease in pregnancy affect the preterm pregnancy rate) remains unaltered.

a) The median survival times among individuals undergoing an isolated aortic valve replacement are just under 1 year for the mechanical valves and just over 1 year for the biological valves. The median survival times among individuals undergoing an isolated mitral valve replacement are around 1 year for those with a mechanical valve and 1.3 years for those with a biological valve. However, as the numbers of patients who remain under follow-up after 1 year are low for both types of valve for isolated aortic and mitral valve replacements, and because it is difficult to read exact values off a graph, these estimates are likely to be unreliable.

b) The authors base their conclusion on the P-values and confidence intervals. Overall, there is no significant association ($P = 0.13$) between the type of valve and mortality (adjusted relative hazard: 0.73), but the 95% confidence interval associated with this is relatively wide, ranging from 0.48 to 1.10 – thus, a biological valve could be up to 52% more protective or 10% less effective than a mechanical valve. Looking at the adjusted hazard ratios for the effect of a biological valve, it appears as if the effect may be stronger if the mitral valve is replaced (adjusted hazard ratio: 0.68, 95% CI: 0.45, 1.53) than if the aortic valve is replaced (adjusted hazard ratio: 0.82, 95% CI: 0.24, 1.93). There is considerable overlap between the confidence intervals, so any difference between the adjusted hazard ratios may be due to chance, and there is no evidence that this difference is real. Therefore, the authors should perform a test for an interaction between the type of valve and the valve location to formally assess whether the impact of valve type varies by the valve location.

c) The P-value for the difference in the proportion of patients with prolonged ventilation between those who received a biological and mechanical valve when undergoing a mitral valve replacement is 0.002, suggesting that this finding is real. However, the authors have performed 32 significance tests in this table alone, of which three are <0.05. A significant effect of prolonged ventilation is entirely consistent with a Type 1 error, and thus it is dangerous to conclude that there is a real difference in the proportion with prolonged ventilation in the two groups.

d) Missing data can, at best, lead to a reduction in study power and, at worst, lead to bias. For this reason, where data are missing, it is preferable to impute these values in some way. The authors chose to use multiple imputation methods to impute the missing values for race, ejection fraction, New York Heart Classification, last creatinine level and predicted risk of mortality to avoid potential bias and/or a reduction in study power. Multiple imputation is one approach to handling missing data. In multiple imputation, the missing values for any variable are predicted using the existing values from other variables to create an imputed data set. A standard statistical analysis is carried out on the imputed data set. This process is performed multiple times, and the results from the different statistical analyses are combined to produce one overall result.

S29

a) The authors chose to use Kaplan–Meier methods and Cox proportional hazards regression models to analyse this data set as they were interested in the time taken for patients to die following transplant; whilst all patients were followed from the same time point (i.e. date of transplant), the calendar date of transplant varied and follow-up on some patients may have been right-censored as they were lost to follow-up. The authors could also have used Poisson regression methods to assess the mortality rate; this approach does not require that all patients are followed for the same period of time and is likely to give similar results to the Cox proportional hazards regression model. Whilst a logistic regression model might also be used to analyse the proportion of patients who died over a specified time period (e.g. one year), this approach would require that all patients be followed for at least one year (i.e. there must be no loss to follow-up before the end of the first year). As this is unlikely to be the case for patients following transplant, such an approach would not be appropriate.

b) As many of the patients in the study died, and as the risk of mortality following transplant is generally highest in the first few days after transplant, the distribution of follow-up times in the study is unlikely to be Normally distributed. Thus, it is preferable to present the median follow-up time rather than the mean follow-up time.

c) At 90 days, and after controlling for differences in donor and recipient status at the time of transplant, it appears that survival rates were 23% higher among those receiving a lung transplant during the night than among those receiving a lung transplant during the day. Whilst the adjusted relative hazard was not statistically significant at 30 days (RH = 1.22, $P = 0.09$), it was significant at 90 days (RH = 1.23, $P = 0.02$). However, there was no effect of the time of day of surgery on 1-year survival (RH = 1.08, $P = 0.19$). Since there is no reason why the effect of time of day

of surgery should have a different impact on survival at 30 days compared to 90 days or 1 year, and as the reported association is in the opposite direction to that suggested by previous studies, it is likely that the significant association at 90 days may have been a Type I error, introduced because of the multiple tests that have been performed on the data set.

d) The P-values shown in the fourth column of Table S29.1 are obtained from the log-rank test. This is a univariable comparison of mortality patterns among those undergoing surgery at different times of day, and does not take account of any differences in the characteristics of patients undergoing transplant. In contrast, the P-values shown in the last column of Table S29.1 are from a Cox proportional hazards regression model in which the authors controlled for any differences in donor and recipient status at the time of transplant.

e) It is assumed that the hazards of mortality are proportional. In other words, if surgery during the daytime is associated with a given increased risk of mortality over the first year, then it should also be associated with this risk over the first 30 and 90 days. The results for the heart transplant recipients appear to suggest that the hazards of mortality are proportional, as the adjusted relative hazard is 1.05 at all three time points. For the lung transplant recipients, however, the adjusted relative hazard changes substantially from 90 days to 1 year, suggesting that the impact of daytime surgery is greatest in the first few months after transplant, but then drops thereafter.

f) For a forwards selection process, the authors start by identifying the variable that contributes most to the fit of the model (based on some criteria of model fit), and then progressively add variables to the model that give the best fit until no further variable significantly improves the fit. For a backwards selection process, the authors start by including all possible variables in their model. They then progressively remove variables from the model that are judged (based on model fit) to be least important. This process continues until none of the remaining variables can be removed without significantly affecting the fit of the model. For this analysis, the authors used a combination of both approaches in a stepwise manner. Whilst this type of procedure removes much of the manual aspect of model selection, it does have several disadvantages. In particular, it is possible that there may be more than one model that fits the data equally well, and the resulting models may not be clinically or biologically sensible. Due to the multiple testing that is involved, this approach is also potentially affected by an increased Type I error rate.

g) The number needed to treat (NNT) during the daytime in the lung transplant group to prevent one death within 90 days is 1 / (difference in absolute risk at 90 days) = 1 / (0.927 − 0.917) = 100. This suggests that 100 patients would have to receive a transplant during the daytime, rather than the night-time, to prevent one death. This is a relatively large figure.

Randomised controlled trial: critical appraisal of Paper 1

A. Title and abstract

1. The trial is identified as a 'Randomized Placebo-Controlled Trial' in the title.
2. The abstract summarises the trial objective, design, methods, results and conclusions.

   The trial design is summarised in the 'Methods' section of the abstract (a randomised, double-blind, placebo-controlled trial).

   The methods are summarised in the 'Methods' section of the abstract (*'Intravenous methylprednisolone (125 gm) was followed by an oral prednisone taper (40 mg for 1 day, 20 mg for 2 days, 10 mg for 3 days, 5 mg for 7 days) versus an identical-appearing placebo regime. All women received promethazine 25 mg and metoclopramide 10 mg intravenously every 6 hours for 24 hours, followed by the same regimen administered orally as needed until discharge'*).

   The results are summarised in the 'Results' section of the abstract (*'56 were randomised to corticosteroids and 54 were administered placebo. Nineteen women in each study group required rehospitalization (34% versus 35%, P = 0.89, for corticosteroids versus placebo, respectively)'*). The conclusions are summarised in the 'Conclusions' section of the abstract (*'the addition of parenteral and oral corticosteroids to the treatment of women with hyperemesis gravidarum did not reduce the need for rehospitalization later in pregnancy'*).

B. Introduction

1. As far as one is able to judge (i.e. without specialist knowledge in the field), the answer to each of these questions is 'yes', as documented in the introductory section of the paper before the 'Materials and Methods' section. In relation to the scientific background, the authors provide details of the percentage of women experiencing hyperemesis gravidarum (3%), the financial burden on the American health system (estimated as $130 million per year), the hours lost from paid work per woman due to nausea and vomiting in early pregnancy (206 hours) and an indication of complications that can arise from hyperemesis gravidarum.

   The authors justify the rationale by explaining that corticosteroids could modify the chemoreceptor trigger zone in the brain that is responsible for nausea and vomiting. They go on to explain that corticosteroids have been used successfully for many years to treat chemotherapy-induced emesis.

   The authors provide a reference (Geiger *et al.*) for a 1959 trial of Bendectin which was shown to be successful for the treatment of nausea and vomiting in pregnancy, but it was removed from the market in 1983 because of claims of teratogenicity. The authors state that, since then, there have been few RCTs to assess different treatment modalities. However, they do not provide any references or indication of the results for these studies, although they do provide the reference for a previous RCT using corticosteroids.

2. The primary aim of the study is indicated in the last sentence of the paragraph before the 'Materials and Methods' section on page 1250 (*'Our goal was to estimate the effect of corticosteroids in reducing the number of women requiring rehospitalization for hyperemesis gravidarum'*). There is no mention of secondary objectives.

C. Methods

1. Trial design

The trial design is described adequately. The women were randomly assigned to receive corticosteroids or placebo (page 1251, paragraph 3, left-hand side (LHS)) in addition to the prevailing treatment. Dose and frequency of corticosteroid treatment are described, as are details of treatment for women with persistent vomiting on day 2 of hospitalisation, diet advice and treatment after discharge (page 1251, paragraph 3, LHS).

a) *Randomisation.* Some but not full details of the randomisation process are provided. The authors explain that randomisation was performed by computer-generated blocks of 20 (page 1251, paragraph 2). No information is given about steps taken to conceal the allocation sequence, and no details are given of the implementation of the randomisation.

b) *Blinding.* The study was described as double-blind (page 1251, paragraph 2, LHS) with both methyl-prednisolone 125 mg and placebo being administered intravenously, followed by a tapering regimen of oral prednisone or an identical appearing placebo. In addition (page 1251, paragraph 3, LHS), both groups of women were provided with crackers and juice on request and were advanced to a regular diet as tolerated. Thus it would appear that both groups of women were treated in the same way and the two regimes appeared identical.

c) *Allocation concealment.* This was not specified.

2. Participants

a) There is a complete description of the eligibility criteria. Eligible patients were those women who complained of nausea and vomiting, previously had not responded to outpatient therapy and demonstrated 3+ or 4+ dipstick urinary ketones as evidence of severe dehydration. Ultrasound was performed on all women to exclude molar pregnancy, confirm a live foetus and establish gestational age. All of this is documented in the last sentence of page 1250 and on page 1252 (paragraph 1, LHS).

b) The women all presented to a particular hospital in Dallas (page 1250, last paragraph, LHS), and the only exclusion criterion was molar pregnancy (page 1251, paragraph 1, LHS). If we can assume that the women in this hospital were reasonably representative of the population of women in the United States, then the study was conducted using an appropriate spectrum of patients.

3. Interventions

a) The intervention for each group is described in sufficient detail. Details are given (page 1251, paragraphs 2 and 3, LHS) of doses of the corticosteroid treatment (i.e. 125 mg intravenously initially and a tapering regimen or oral prednisone, 40 mg for 1 day, 20 mg for 3 days, 10 mg for 3 days and 5 mg for 7 days). Women with persistent vomiting on day 2 received an additional 80 mg dose. Women in the placebo arm received similar placebo treatment at all stages.

b) The groups were treated in similar fashion. All the women were provided with the prevailing treatment for persistent hyperemesis gravidarum. Details are given on the LHS of page 1251, paragraph 2. After treatment, all women were provided with crackers and juice on request and were advanced to a regular diet as tolerated (page 1251, paragraph 3, LHS). Each woman was counselled by a nutritionalist before discharge (page 1251, paragraph 3, LHS). At discharge all women were treated with the same additional therapy as needed, and this treatment approach was used for women requiring readmission for hyperemesis gravidarum (page 1251, paragraph 3, LHS). All women underwent the same battery of laboratory tests (page 1251, paragraph 4, LHS).

4. Outcomes

a) Consideration is given to all the important outcomes. In addition to the proportion of women needing rehospitalisation later in the pregnancy (the primary outcome), a number of other outcomes are described, for example number of ER visits, number of days in hospital for the first admission and total number of days in hospital for all admissions (Table 3), as well as pregnancy complications (Table 4) and neonatal outcomes (Table 5). Without specialist knowledge in the field, we can only assume that these constitute all the important outcomes.

b) The primary outcome (the number of women requiring rehospitalisation for hyperemesis gravidarum) is clearly defined (page 1250, paragraph 2, right-hand side (RHS) and page 1253, paragraph 1, LHS). The results relating to the secondary outcomes, as listed in Section 3d(i), are described, but the secondary outcomes are not formally described as such in the paper.

c) There do not appear to be any changes to the outcomes after the trial started.

5. Sample size

a) There is a power statement to justify the overall sample size (page 1251, paragraph 2, RHS). This power statement does not indicate the form of statistical analysis on which it is based (i.e. there is no mention of the Chi-squared test) although it is clear that it relates to a comparison of percentages. The power statement does specify the values of all the factors that affect sample size. In particular, the authors state that a power of 80% for a two-sided test with a significance level of 0.05 was used for the sample size calculation to detect a reduction in the number of women needing rehospitalisation from 30% to 5%.

b) There were no interim analyses.

c) There were no subgroup analyses.

6. Statistical methods

a) A list of the statistical methods used to compare groups is provided (page 125, paragraph 2, LHS), although the paper says *'statistical analysis included'*, possibly suggesting that there were other statistical techniques that were used that were not listed. The three tests listed are the Chi-squared test, Student *t*-test and Wilcoxon signed-rank test. The paper does not explain the circumstances in which each test was used. The Chi-squared test would have been used to compare relevant percentages for categorical data. The paper does not define the Student *t*-test explicitly so it could be the two-sample *t*-test comparing independent groups (i.e. the treatment and placebo groups) or the paired *t*-test comparing numerical outcomes in dependent groups (i.e. before and after treatment in the same individual). The Wilcoxon signed-rank test is used to compare numerical outcomes in dependent groups when the assumption of Normality of the paired differences is not satisfied so that the paired *t*-test is not appropriate. However, the results of any paired comparisons are not included, so it is not clear when the Wilcoxon signed-rank test would have been employed.

b) There is no mention of checking the assumptions underlying the Chi-squared test or the *t*-test.

c) There were no additional analyses.

D. Results

1. Participant numbers and dates

a) There is a participant flow chart (Figure 1) showing the number of women eligible, assigned to each treatment arm, lost to follow up in each group and analysed.

b) There were 16 women who were lost to follow-up, eight in each treatment arm (page 1251, paragraph 4, RHS). No reasons are given for the losses to follow-up. However, these women were described as not significantly different from the remainder of the cohort with respect to maternal characteristics, laboratory tests and course before randomisation (page 1251, paragraph 4, RHS).

c) Dates of recruitment are provided: from July 6, 1998 to August 22, 2001 (page 1250, paragraph 3, RHS). All women were followed up until the end of their pregnancies as it is stated (page 1251, paragraph 4, RHS) that the 110 women in the study (i.e. excluding the 16 lost to follow-up) were delivered at Parkland Hospital.

2. Baseline data

a) Table 1 shows the baseline demographic and clinical characteristics for each group. Table 2 shows the laboratory characteristics for each group.

b) It would appear that there is no difference between the two groups with respect to any of the characteristics in Tables 1 and 2 when informally comparing the means and standard deviations for the numerical variables and the percentages for the categorical variables. The paper provides a P-value for each of these comparisons, indicating that a hypothesis test has been performed in each instance. It should be noted that it is not appropriate to perform a hypothesis test to establish whether or not randomisation has worked (i.e. whether it has produced comparable groups) because a hypothesis test is used to assess if the difference between the two groups could be due to chance. The groups are constructed by random (i.e. chance) allocation in a RCT so that the difference between baseline values must be due to chance. Any P-values <0.05 are likely, therefore, to reflect Type I errors.

3. Numbers analysed

a) The ITT analysis is specified in paragraph 4 on the RHS of page 1251. The ITT analysis is appropriate in that the available data were analysed according to the manner in which the women were actually treated. As there were no known protocol deviations (including any losses to follow-up), the ITT approach would produce identical results to the per protocol approach.

b) There were no protocol deviations. There is a statement indicating that there were no cross-overs and that the same study drug assignment was used in women who were readmitted (page 1251, paragraph 3, LHS).

4. Outcomes of interest

a) *Main outcome of interest.* The primary outcome variable is the number of women requiring rehospitalisation. It is shown in Table 3 that 19/56 (34%) in the corticosteroid group and 19/54 (35%) in the placebo group required rehospitalisation. These percentages are also provided in paragraph 1 on the LHS of page 1253. The authors indicate in Table 3 that the percentages are not significantly different ($P = 0.89$).

b) *Magnitude of the effect of interest.* There is no indication of the magnitude of the effect of interest. For this study, the most relevant effect of interest is the difference in the percentages requiring rehospitalisation in the two groups (i.e. it is 33.9% − 35.2% = −1.3%).

c) *Precision of the effect of interest.* There is no indication of the precision of the effect of interest, which is not surprising given that no estimate is provided of the effect of interest. In fact, the difference in the percentages requiring rehospitalisation in the corticosteroid and placebo groups (the effect of interest) is estimated as 33.9% − 35.2% = −1.3%, its estimated standard error is 9.07% and the 95% CI for the true difference in the percentages is −19.1% to 16.5%.

5. Additional analyses
There were no additional analyses. However, there are a number of variables other than those relating to the primary aim that were analysed. Means (accompanied by standard deviations rather than standard errors of the mean or CIs) and percentages are provided for these secondary variables as well as P-values resulting from any hypothesis tests performed (Tables 3, 4 and 5).

6. Harms
All important harms in each group are documented. Table 4 shows the frequencies and percentages of the mothers' complications, and Table 5 shows the frequencies and percentages for adverse neonatal outcomes.

E. Discussion

1. Deciding whether the results are important

a) The key findings are summarised in the 'Discussion' section (beginning of paragraph 1 on the LHS of page 1253) and in the Abstract.

b) There is no reason to suppose that the results do not make biological sense even though the authors were disappointed with them (page 1253, paragraph 1, LHS). The effect of interest is not provided in the paper, but the differences in the percentages requiring rehospitalisation in the corticosteroid and placebo groups have been calculated as −1.3% with a 95% CI of −19.1% to 16.5% (see D4 (b) and (c)). If the true difference in the percentages requiring hospitalisation is equal to −19.1% (i.e. the lower limit of the 95% CI), this would represent an important benefit for corticosteroids and suggests that their use should be advocated. However, the upper limit of the 95% CI is 16.5%, in which case the use of the placebo is substantially better than that of corticosteroids. The conclusions drawn from interpreting the upper and lower limits of the 95% confidence interval for the difference in the percentages are diametrically opposite, indicating that the conclusion (that there is no evidence that corticosteroids when compared to placebo are effective in reducing rehospitalisation for hyperemesis gravidarum) is correct.

c) There is no evaluation of the numbers needed to treat, but this would not be relevant since there was no evidence of a difference between the two treatments for the primary outcome.

2. Limitations
The discussion of trial limitations is restricted to the possibly inadequate sample size (the end of paragraph 1 on the LHS of page 1253). The authors suggest that the sample size might be too small because it was based on an overly optimistic improvement in the primary outcome from 30% to 5%.

3. Generalisability
There is no discussion of the generalisability of the trial findings.

4. Interpretation
The interpretation of the trial findings is consistent with the results, after taking the benefits and harms into consideration. The authors correctly state in the final paragraph of the paper that their results support the conclusion of Magee

et al., whose pooled results failed to show that corticosteroids reduced the number of readmissions to hospital for hyperemesis gravidarum. Expressing the conclusion in this way is more correct than stating (as in the abstract) that the corticosteroid treatment did not reduce the need for rehospitalisation later in pregnancy in view of the possible small sample size and consequent low power. It should be remembered, as stated by Altman and Bland (1995), that 'absence of evidence is not evidence of absence'.

F. Other information

1. **Registration**   The trial was not registered, but this was not strongly advocated in 2003 when the paper was published.
2. **Protocol**   There is no information about where the protocol can be accessed, but this was not strongly advocated in 2003 when the paper was published.
3. **Funding**   The sources of funding are not documented, but this was not strongly advocated in 2003 when the paper was published.
4. **Conflict of interest**   No information is provided.

Reference

Altman DG, Bland JM. Absence of evidence is not evidence of absence. *BMJ* (1995), 311: 485.

Observational study: critical appraisal of Paper 2

A. Title and abstract

1. The study is identified as a *'Multicenter Prospective Study'* in the title. This does not, however, identify the study design as a cohort (interventional studies are also prospective).

2. The abstract summarises the study design, methods, results and conclusions.

    The study design and inclusion criteria are identified in the 'Methods' section of the abstract: *'We acquired data from a multicenter prospective cohort that included 3322 consecutive patients undergoing major digestive surgery across 47 different facilities'*. The authors then state that *'A multivariate analysis was used to identify the independent risk factors of mortality in elderly patients (n = 1796)'*. Note that the exact type of statistical analysis is not specified. Furthermore, the term 'multivariate' strictly refers to an analysis of two or more outcomes that are investigated simultaneously (which is not the case here) and is therefore misleading. Use of the term 'multivariable' is preferable. *'The end-point was defined as 30-day postoperative mortality'*, and the authors stated that they assessed 27 pre-, intra- and postoperative demographic and clinical variables.

    The overall mortality rate among elderly patients ($\geq$65 years old) was 10.6%; in elderly patients, risk factors for mortality identified in the abstract are age $\geq$85 years, emergency surgery, anaemia, white cell count >10000/mm^3, American Association of Anesthesiologists (ASA) class IV and a palliative cancer operation, with odds ratios and 95% confidence intervals provided for each.

    In the 'Conclusion' section of the abstract, the authors state that *'Characterization of independent validated risk indicators for mortality in elderly patients undergoing major digestive surgery is essential and may lead to an efficient specific workup, which constitutes a necessary step to developing a dedicated score for elderly patients'*. No specific limitations are mentioned.

B. Introduction

1. The introductory section on page 375 is relatively brief. The authors note that life expectancy has steadily increased in recent decades and, as a result, the number of major surgical operations offered to elderly patients has also risen. They point out that postoperative mortality in this group remains high and that guidance on the most appropriate management of this group depends on validated outcome indicators, for which information is lacking. The authors provide a large number of references to support their claims. They also explain that previous studies have focussed on a particular disease, a specific operation or an arbitrarily defined age group, and they are not consistent with regard to definitions and other matters.

2. The primary objective of the study is to identify risk factors for postoperative mortality in patients aged 65 years and older, using young patients as a control group (page 375, paragraph 2, LHS). No secondary objectives are defined. There is no mention of modifications of the original protocol.

C. Methods

1. **Study design** The two authors describe the study design in the final paragraph of the introductory section on page 375 (*'the study is based on a prospective multicenter cohort of 3322 consecutive patients undergoing major digestive surgery'*). In the second paragraph of the 'Patients and Methods' section on page 375, they provide details of the cohort: whilst the full cohort had an age range of 16–99 years, 1796 (54%) patients who were over 65 years of age were the group of particular interest for this study. In the next paragraph, the authors also describe the setting of the study and the dates of surgery (i.e. the dates of recruitment for the study): *'Patients underwent surgery between January 01, 2002 and December 31, 2004 in 47 French surgical centers (17 universities [53% of the patients], 27 general [37% of the patients], and 3 private hospitals [10% of the patients]). The average number of patients enrolled by center was 75 ± 63 (median 49, range 0–362).'* The authors also note that *'A minimum enrollment of 30 patients per year was necessary for a facility to participate in our study'*, although it is noteworthy that the lower limit of the quoted range indicates that at least one centre did not recruit any patients. The 47 surgical centres are not listed, but some information on this topic can be gleaned from the Appendix.

2. **Participants**

    a) Eligibility criteria are provided in the last paragraph of page 375 and at the top of page 376: *'eligibility criteria included patients over the age of 16 who underwent a major digestive operation (defined as "major or major plus" according to Copeland or "complex grade 3, 4, and 5" according to Aust et al.) as well as certain other operations (intraperitoneal hyperthermic chemotherapy, bariatric surgery bypass, and strictureplasty)'*. Although the initial patient cohort comprised 3881 individuals (page 376, paragraph 1, LHS), patients who had not been followed up (but were not known to have died) within the first 30 days were excluded ($n = 308$) from the initial cohort as were those with missing data on three or more of the factors of interest ($n = 251$). Thus the cohort described in the paper (the 'study cohort') comprised 3322 individuals (=3881 − 308 − 251). Patients were consecutively seen within each participating clinic.

    b) Not applicable – this is a cohort study.

    c) No information is provided on how the cohort was followed up, although it is assumed that this is through routine clinical monitoring (at least over the first 30 days after surgery).

d) It is stated in the first sentence of the 'Patients and Methods' section on page 375 that the patients who underwent major digestive surgery were consecutively recruited. Since the cohort therefore encompasses all potential patients in the study centres, each of which required a minimum enrolment of 30 patients per year, we can assume that the study was conducted using an appropriate spectrum of patients.

e) Not applicable – the study was not matched.

3. Variables

a) The primary outcome was mortality during the first 30 days after surgery (page 375, 'Patients and Methods' section, paragraph 3).

   The choice of potential exposures and predictors is based on three previously published studies. A total of 27 demographic and clinical variables were considered (listed in paragraph 1 of the 'Risk Factors' section on page 376), all of which had been reported to be associated with surgery outcomes. These included age (≥ 65 or <65 years), which was the primary exposure of interest. A definition is provided for each covariate.

b) Other than providing a definition of the covariates to be collected, no information is provided on the comparability of the variables across the 47 different participating centres.

4. Bias   No mention is made of bias in the 'Patients and Methods' section.

5. Sample size   No justification is provided for the sample size.

6. Statistical methods

a) Almost all of the potential continuous covariates were dichotomised prior to analysis. No justification is provided for the choice of threshold that was used to dichotomise each covariate, although it is assumed that this follows earlier published analyses.

b) For the primary analysis (identification of risk factors), the authors utilised a multivariable logistic regression analysis with mortality as the outcome (page 376, 'Statistical Analysis' section, paragraph 4). Factors that were associated with the outcome ($P < 0.10$) in univariate analyses were included in the multivariable regression model; a forwards stepwise elimination method was used to identify covariates in the final model. The final model was applied separately to older (≥ 65 years) and younger (<65 years) patients. In the penultimate paragraph of the 'Statistical Analysis' section, the authors state that 'a post estimation of the model goodness of fit was performed using the C index and Hosmer–Lemeshow tests. A bootstrapping procedure with 200 replications was used to assess the stability of the model'.

c) As described in Section C6(b), the final model was applied separately to the subgroups comprising older and younger patients.

d) As described in C2(a), patients who had not been followed up (but were not known to have died) within the first 30 days were excluded from the initial cohort as were those with missing data on three or more of the factors of interest. No further exclusions were applied. The authors describe their methods for dealing with missing covariate data in the penultimate paragraph of the 'Statistical Analysis' section on page 376 ('The missing values were treated according to an imputation procedure'), although no further details, including the precise method of imputation or the number of data sets imputed, are provided.

e) As noted in Section C2(a), patients who had not been followed up (but were not known to have died) within the first 30 days were excluded from the initial cohort ($n = 308$); no further losses to follow-up occurred.

f) No sensitivity analyses were performed.

D. Results

1. Participant numbers and dates

a) As noted in C2(a), patients with insufficient follow-up within 30 days post-operation and with missing data on more than three of the covariates were excluded from the initial cohort of 3881 patients (page 376, paragraph 1, LHS). Since they were therefore not part of the study cohort, no further information is provided on these patients. No flow chart is provided.

b) Those who were excluded were excluded due to lack of follow-up data within 30 days post-operation or due to missing covariate data (page 376, paragraph 1, LHS).

2. Descriptive data

a) Table 1 provides a full description of the characteristics of the younger and older cohorts (although not the combined cohort). By splitting the patients into the younger and older cohorts, it is possible to identify factors that may differ between the two cohorts; the authors provide P-values for all comparisons of the older and younger cohorts, with those that are significant ($P \leq 0.05$ in this case) highlighted in bold. These P-values are not adjusted to make allowance for the large number of tests that have been performed (Table 1 has 33 such comparisons).

b) The level of missing data is, rather confusingly, summarised at the foot of Table 1, with the mean, median and range of the number of patients with missing data per variable quoted. Thus, on average (based on the mean), 75 patients had missing data on each variable, although this number ranged from 0 to 422. Note that the values in the text ('42/1484' and '191/1605') relate to the mortality rates rather than the missing data.

c) Although total follow-up times are not provided, the period of primary interest in this study is the first 30 days post-surgery. As all patients are followed for at least this time, the follow-up time is summarised, and information on longer term follow-up is of limited relevance.

3. Main results

a) *Main outcome measures.* As reported in the first paragraph of the 'Results' section on page 376, 233 (7%) of the study cohort died within the first 30 days post-operation (no confidence interval is provided for the overall mortality rate). Mortality rates are depicted graphically, stratified by age group, in Figure 1, although the number of deaths in each age stratum is not provided.

b) *Magnitude of effects of interest.* In the study cohort, being older than 65 years was a significant risk factor for mortality (page 376, 'Results', paragraph 1) with an unadjusted odds ratio of 2.21 ($P = 0.0001$).

   Univariate (unadjusted) estimates of the odds ratio of death (30 days) for each of the 27 potential risk factors, separately for those <65 years and ≥65 years, are shown in Table 3, with adjusted estimates provided in Table 4.

   In the text (page 376, 'Results' section), the authors present selected confounder adjusted estimates of interest. They state that *'being older than 65 was on its own a significant independent risk factor of mortality (OR, 2.21: 95% CI, 1.36 – 3.59: P = 001)'*. This appears to be the only information reported from the initial multivariable logistic regression analysis on the study cohort. The authors also extract some information from the tables. For example (from Table 4), they indicate that among those aged ≥65 years, being aged ≥85 years was (not surprisingly) associated with an increased mortality rate, with an odds ratio of 2.62 ($P = 0.32$), and (from Table 2) *'The mortality after emergency procedures in elderly patients was 33.5% (102 of 304) versus 7.4% (12 of 162) in young patients (P ≤ 0.001)'*.

   In addition, in the first paragraph of the 'Results' section on page 376, the authors describe the relationship between age (group) and mortality as *'postoperative mortality = 0.002 × exp (0.63 × age)'* – the parameter estimates from this model provide an estimate of the association between age and mortality in the study cohort. However, the authors do not assess the appropriateness of this model by using formal statistical procedures and do not provide a P-value to support it. Furthermore, it is not clear from the 'Statistical Analysis' section whether age has been incorporated into this regression model as a continuous covariate (i.e. per year) or after stratification into the different age groups.

c) *Precision of effects of interest.* 95% confidence intervals are provided in the first paragraph of the 'Results' section on page 376 for the overall odds ratio of death for age >65 years (1.36 to 3.59) and for all odds ratios reported in Tables 3 and 4.

d) As noted in Section C6(b), covariates were selected for initial inclusion in the multivariable model if they were associated ($P < 0.10$) with mortality in univariate analyses. These covariates are detailed in Table 3, separately for the two age groups. Factors were then selected for inclusion in the final multivariable model using a forwards stepwise selection procedure.

4. Other analyses

Although the authors identified risk factors for mortality in the older and younger cohorts separately, no formal tests of interaction were performed to assess whether any differences in mortality for these risk factors between the two cohorts were likely to be real. No sensitivity analyses were performed.

E. Discussion

1. Summary of key results

a) Although the main findings are reported on page 377 in the 'Discussion', this occurs over the first eight paragraphs or so. Thus, it is questionable whether the authors have truly 'summarised' the main results. It would have been helpful for the key findings to be summarised in a single, short paragraph.

b) Given the very large number of factors considered, it is unclear whether any of the statistically significant associations are likely to reflect Type 1 errors. However, all factors were initially selected on the basis that they had been reported to be associated with mortality in other published studies. Thus, these results appear to make biological sense and should be seen as confirmatory rather than exploratory, although with reservations because of the problem of multiple testing.

c) For the overall analysis of the impact of age (>65) on mortality, the 95% confidence interval ranged from 1.36 to 3.59, suggesting that the odds of mortality in the older group could be anything from 36% to 259% higher than that in the younger group. Whilst this is a wide confidence interval, it is likely that the impact of older age would be regarded as clinically important, regardless of whether the true value took the lower or upper limit of this range.

   Confidence intervals for some of the reported associations in the younger and older age cohorts were very wide (Table 4): for example, among the younger cohort, severe medical complications were associated with a 108-fold greater odds of mortality, with the 95% confidence interval ranging from around 9 to almost 14 000! Among the older cohort, associations with some of the factors had confidence intervals that could be interpreted as ambiguous. For example, for white cell count >10 000/mm^3, if the lower limit of the confidence interval (1.08) represented the true value of the effect, the observed effect would possibly not be viewed as clinically important. If, however, the upper limit of the confidence interval (3.35) represented the true value of the effect, the effect would be deemed to be clinically important as this would suggest a more than threefold greater odds of mortality. The perceived importance of this finding is therefore not clear, and the results may be interpreted as ambiguous.

d) The authors do not provide this information.

2. Limitations

The authors note three potential limitations of their study (page 380, 'Discussion', penultimate paragraph) including a lack of information on some potentially important markers (particularly nutritional status, frailty or pre-frailty markers) and the possibility of selection bias introduced by the type of patient who is offered (or agrees to) major surgery. Other limitations, for example, bias introduced by multiple testing, missing data or imprecisions in data collection, are not discussed.

3. **Generalisability**   Other than discussion of potential selection bias (mentioned in E2), no further discussion on generalisability is provided.

4. **Interpretation**   The authors performed a large number of statistical tests; no attempt was made to adjust the P-values from these tests to take account of multiple testing. However, as the study was established to potentially validate findings from other published studies, rather than to identify and explore new associations, the study findings are discussed in a reasonably cautious manner.

F. Other information

1. **Funding**   The source of funding for this cohort study is stated on page 375 (LHS), but the role of the funders is not described.

2. **Conflict of interest**   No conflict of interest statements are provided, although it is difficult to see how any conflict of interest could have a major impact on the results.

Appendices
Appendix I: list of multiple-choice questions with relevant chapter numbers from *Medical Statistics at a Glance* (3rd edn) and associated topics

Handling data

M1. Chapters 1, 2, 5 (types of variables, averages)

M2. Chapter 1 (types of variables)

M3. Chapter 2 (data entry)

M4. Chapter 2 (data entry, dates, coded questions)

M5. Chapter 3 (data entry, checking for errors)

M6. Chapter 3 (outliers)

M7. Chapter 4 (diagrams)

M8. Chapters 4, 7 (shape of distribution, Normal distribution)

M9. Chapter 4 (pie chart, bar chart, histogram, skewness, box plot)

M10. Chapters 5, 6 (measures of location and spread)

M11. Chapters 5, 9 (median, geometric mean, logarithmic transformation)

M12. Chapters 5, 6 (measures of location and spread, reference ranges)

M13. Chapters 5, 6 (percentiles, averages, spread)

M14. Chapter 7 (Normal distribution)

M15. Chapter 8 (Binomial, Poisson, Chi-squared and Lognormal distributions)

M16. Chapters 1, 7, 9, 17 (transformations, Normal distribution)

M17. Chapter 9 (transformations)

Sampling and estimation

M18. Chapter 10 (sampling distribution of the mean)

M19. Chapters 5, 6, 7, 10, 11 (spread, Normal distribution, sampling distributions)

M20. Chapters 11, 15 (confidence intervals, cohort studies)

M21. Chapter 11 (confidence interval for the mean)

Study design

M22. Chapters 12, 15 (cohort studies, association)

M23. Chapter 12 (assessing causality)

M24. Chapters 13, 14 (randomised controlled trials (RCTs), cross-over trials)

M25. Chapters 13, 14 (RCTs, composite endpoints)

M26. Chapters 13, 33 (factorial, cross-over, parallel and completely randomised designs, interaction, statistical interaction)

M27. Chapters 12, 14 (cluster randomised trials, sample size, unit of investigation)

M28. Chapter 14 (clinical trials, randomisation, sequential studies)

M29. Chapters 13, 15, 16 (cohort studies, outcomes, recall bias)

M30. Chapter 15 (cohort studies)

M31. Chapters 12, 15, 16 (case–control studies, risk, relative risk, odds ratio)

M32. Chapters 12, 16 (experimental studies, case–control studies, relative risk)

M33. Chapters 12, 16, 29, 30 (case–control studies, odds ratio, logistic regression, multiple linear regression)

Hypothesis testing

M34. Chapters 11, 17 (hypothesis tests, confidence intervals, bio-equivalence trials, nonparametric tests)

M35. Chapters 18, 20 (paired tests, multiple comparisons, Bonferroni correction)

M36. Chapter 18 (Type I and II errors in hypothesis testing, significance level)

Basic techniques for analysing data

Numerical data

M37. Chapters 4, 19 (shape of distribution, one-sample t-test)

M38. Chapter 19 (one-sample t-test, sign test)

M39. Chapters 5, 12, 20 (averages, Wilcoxon signed-ranks test, need for a control)

M40. Chapters 19, 20, 21 (analysis of paired numerical data, Wilcoxon signed-ranks test, paired and unpaired t-tests)

M41. Chapters 20, 21, 22 (paired and unpaired t-tests, one-way analysis of variance (ANOVA))

M42. Chapters 20, 21 (Wilcoxon signed-ranks test, Mann–Whitney U-test, unpaired t-test)

M43. Chapter 22 (one-way ANOVA)

Categorical data

M44. Chapters 7, 20, 23, 24 (Binomial and Normal distributions, Wilcoxon signed-ranks test, hypothesis test on a single proportion, Fisher's exact test, Chi-squared test)

M45. Chapters 11, 23 (confidence intervals, testing a single proportion)

M46. Chapters 24, 30 (Chi-squared test, logistic regression)

M47. Chapter 24 (comparing two proportions, Chi-squared test)

M48. Chapters 15, 24, 25 (cohort studies, Fisher's exact test, 2×2 tables, Chi-squared test with more than with two categories)

M49. Chapters 24, 25 (associations in an $r \times c$ contingency table, Chi-squared test, McNemar's test)

Regression and correlation

M50. Chapters 4, 26 (skewed distributions, Pearson correlation coefficient)

M51. Chapter 26 (Pearson correlation coefficient)

M52. Chapter 27 (assumptions underlying linear regression)

M53. Chapter 28 (linear regression, scaling)

M54. Chapter 28 (linear regression, goodness of fit, centring, scaling, influential points)

M55. Chapter 29 (multiple linear regression)

M56. Chapter 29 (multiple linear regression, collinearity)

M57. Chapters 29, 30, 34 (multiple linear regression, logistic regression, confounding, odds ratio)

M58. Chapter 10 (logistic regression, odds, model Chi-square, deviance)

M59. Chapter 31 (rates)

Medical Statistics at a Glance Workbook, First Edition. Aviva Petrie and Caroline Sabin.
© 2013 Aviva Petrie and Caroline Sabin. Published 2013 by Blackwell Publishing Ltd. **117**

M60. Chapters 13, 31, 34 (stratification, Poisson regression, relative rates, interaction, stratification)

M61. Chapters 9, 31, 33 (transformations, Poisson regression, relative rates)

M62. Chapters 31, 34 (Poisson regression, relative rates, confounding)

M63. Chapter 31 (Poisson regression, extra-Poisson variation)

M64. Chapter 32 (generalised linear model, method of least squares, maximum likelihood estimation, likelihood, link function)

M65. Chapter 13 (explanatory variables in statistical models, confounding, effect modification, over-fitting)

Important considerations

M66. Chapter 34 (bias, confounding)

M67. Chapter 35 (checking assumptions, sensitivity analysis)

M68. Chapter 36 (sample size estimation, power, significance level)

M69. Chapters 35, 36 (robust estimation, sample size estimation, power, significance level, pilot studies)

M70. Chapter 37 (presenting results, CONSORT statement, STROBE statement, QUORUM statement)

Additional techniques

M71. Chapter 18 (diagnostic tests, area under the curve (AUC))

M72. Chapter 38 (diagnostic tests, sensitivity, specificity, positive predictive value, negative predictive value, likelihood)

M73. Chapter 39 (assessing agreement for a categorical variable, Cohen's kappa)

M74. Chapters 26, 39 (correlation, assessing agreement for categorical and numerical variables, Cohen's kappa, intra-class correlation coefficient, Bland and Altman diagram)

M75. Chapter 40 (evidence-based medicine (EBM), hierarchy of evidence, number needed to treat (NNT))

M76. Chapter 41 (clustered data)

M77. Chapter 41 (clustered data, repeated measurements)

M78. Chapter 42 (analysis of hierarchical data, random effects model, intra-class correlation coefficient)

M79. Chapter 43 (meta-analysis, odds ratios, forest plot, publication bias)

M80. Chapter 43 (meta-analysis, systematic review, random effect, I^2, publication bias)

M81. Chapters 29, 44 (choice of reference category, survival analysis, hazard ratio)

M82. Chapter 44 (survival analysis, censoring, hazard ratio, log rank test)

M83. Chapter 45 (Bayesian analysis, likelihood, prior, diagnostic tests)

M84. Chapter 46 (prognostic scores, area under the receiver operating characteristic (AUROC) curve, goodness of fit)

M85. Chapter 46 (prognostic scores, receiver operating characteristic (ROC) curve, bootstrapping, goodness of fit)

Appendices Appendix I: list of multiple-choice questions with relevant chapter numbers from *Medical Statistics at a Glance* (3rd edn) and

118 associated topics

Appendix II: list of structured questions with relevant chapter numbers from *Medical Statistics at a Glance* (3rd edn) and associated topics

S1. Chapters 1, 2, 3, 4 (type of data, data entry, error checking and outliers, displaying data graphically)

S2. Chapters 5, 6, 11 (mean, standard deviation (SD), standard error of the mean (SEM), confidence intervals, median)

S3. Chapters 5, 6, 17, 21, 24, 26 (summarising data, transformations, *P*-value, comparing numerical and categorical data in two groups, Fisher's exact test, correlation)

S4. Chapters 5, 6, 16, 30, 34 (summarising data, study design, logistic regression, odds ratios)

S5. Chapter 14 (randomised controlled trials, intention to treat and per-protocol analysis, generalizability)

S6. Chapters 18, 36 (Type I and II errors in hypothesis testing, power and significance level, sample size calculations)

S7. Chapter 20 (paired *t*-test, confidence intervals)

S8. Chapters 20, 25, 34 (comparing categorical data in more than two groups, Chi-squared test, comparing numerical data when data are not independent, bias, nonresponders)

S9. Chapters 4, 5, 21, 34 (summarising data, Normal distribution, displaying data graphically, Mann–Whitney *U*-test, Wilcoxon rank-sum test, randomisation, bias)

S10. Chapters 22, 34 (one-way analysis of variance (ANOVA), *post-hoc* multiple comparison tests, causation, bias)

S11. Chapter 24 (Chi-squared test, contingency tables)

S12. Chapters 25, 30, 34 (comparing categorical data in more than two groups, logistic regression, bias, test for trend)

S13. Chapters 26, 27, 28 (correlation, simple linear regression)

S14. Chapters 29, 33 (multiple linear regression, explanatory variables)

S15. Chapters 30, 44 (binary outcomes, logistic regression, odds ratios, survival analysis)

S16. Chapters 6, 15, 28, 31, 33 (percentiles, scaling, rates, incidence rate ratios, Poisson regression, cohort studies, explanatory variables)

S17. Chapters 31, 33, 34 (rates, incidence rate ratios, Poisson regression, bias, interaction)

S18. Chapters 31, 33, 34, 42 (rates, incidence rate ratios, Poisson regression, explanatory variables, causal pathway, clustered data)

S19. Chapter 34 (bias and confounding, random and systematic errors)

S20. Chapters 34, 41, 42 (clustered data, confounding, random- or mixed-effects models)

S21. Chapters, 21, 24, 35 (checking assumptions, *t*-tests, Fisher's exact test)

S22. Chapters 21, 36 (*t*-tests, sample size estimation, power)

S23. Chapter 38 (diagnostic tests, sensitivity, specificity, negative predictive value (NPV), positive predictive value (PPV), receiver operating characteristic (ROC) curves, likelihood ratios)

S24. Chapters 38, 46 (diagnostic scores, prognostic scores, area under the receiver operating characteristic (AUROC) curve, sensitivity, specificity, PPV, NPV)

S25. Chapter 39 (assessing agreement for a categorical variable, Cohen's kappa)

S26. Chapters 26, 39 (correlation, measuring agreement, Bland and Altman diagram, limits of agreement, British Standards Institution repeatability coefficient)

S27. Chapters 16, 43 (odds ratios, meta-analysis, I^2, funnel plot, fixed-effects analysis)

S28. Chapters 3, 18, 33, 34, 44 (missing values, Type I error and multiple testing, interaction, confounding, survival analysis)

S29. Chapters 18, 34, 40, 44 (multiple testing, number needed to treat (NNT), confounding, Cox regression model, Kaplan–Meier survival analysis, confounding)

Appendix III: chapter numbers from *Medical Statistics at a Glance* (3rd edn) with relevant multiple-choice questions and structured questions

Chapter	Multiple-choice question(s)	Structured question(s)	Chapter	Multiple-choice question(s)	Structured question(s)
1. Types of data	1, 2, 16	1	24. Categorical data: two proportions	46, 47, 44, 48, 49	3, 8, 11, 21
2. Data entry	1, 3, 4	1	25. Categorical data: more than two categories	48, 49	8, 12
3. Error checking and outliers	5, 6	1, 28	26. Correlation	50, 51, 74	3, 13, 26
4. Displaying data diagrammatically	7, 8, 9, 37, 50	1, 9	27. The theory of linear regression	52	13
5. Describing data: the 'average'	1, 10, 11, 12, 13, 19, 39	2, 3, 4, 9	28. Performing a linear regression analysis	53, 54	13, 16
6. Describing data: the 'spread'	10, 12, 13, 19	2, 3, 4, 16	29. Multiple linear regression	33, 55, 56, 57, 81	14
7. Theoretical distributions: the Normal distribution	8, 14, 16, 19, 44	–	30. Binary outcomes and logistic regression	33, 46, 57, 58	4, 12, 15
8. Theoretical distributions: other distributions	15, 44	–	31. Rates and Poisson regression	59, 60, 61, 62, 63	16, 17, 18, 29
9. Transformations	11, 16, 17, 61	3	32. Generalized linear models	64	–
10. Sampling and sampling distributions	18, 19	–	33. Explanatory variables in statistical models	26, 60, 61, 65	14, 16, 17, 18, 28
11. Confidence intervals	19, 20, 21, 34, 45	2	34. Bias and confounding	57, 60, 62, 66	4, 8, 9, 10, 12, 17, 18, 19, 20, 28, 29
12. Study design I	22, 23, 27, 31, 32, 33, 39	–	35. Checking assumptions	67, 69	21
13. Study design II	24, 25, 26, 29, 60	–	36. Sample size calculations	68, 69	6, 22
14. Clinical trials	24, 25, 27, 28	5	37. Presenting results	70	–
15. Cohort studies	20, 22, 29, 30, 31, 48	16	38. Diagnostic tools	71, 72	23, 24
16. Case–control studies	29, 31, 32, 33	4, 27	39. Assessing agreement	73, 74	25, 26
17. Hypothesis testing	16, 24	3	40. Evidence-based medicine	75	29
18. Errors in hypothesis testing	35, 36	6, 28, 29	41. Methods for clustered data	76, 77	20
19. Numerical data: a single group	37, 38, 40	–	42. Regression models for clustered data	78	18, 20
20. Numerical data: two related groups	39, 40, 35, 41, 42	7, 8	43. Systematic reviews and meta-analysis	79, 80	27
21. Numerical data: two unrelated groups	40, 41, 42	3, 9, 21, 22	44. Survival analysis	81, 82	15, 28, 29
22. Numerical data: more than two groups	43	10	45. Bayesian methods	83	–
23. Categorical data: a single proportion	44, 45	–	46. Developing prognostic scores	84, 85	24

Medical Statistics at a Glance Workbook, First Edition. Aviva Petrie and Caroline Sabin.